I Had This
Little Cancer...

————————————

I Had This Little Cancer...

JEAN PRADEAU

Translated by June P. Wilson

ABELARD-SCHUMAN   NEW YORK

10 9 8 7 6 5 4 3 2 1

Library of Congress Cataloging in Publication Data

Pradeau, Jean.
    I had this little cancer. . .

    Translation of Un petit truc de rien du tout.
      1. Cancer—Personal narratives. 2. Pradeau, Jean.
I. Title.
RC263.P713   362.1′9′699409 [B]   76-3567
ISBN 0-200-04036-7

I Had This
Little Cancer...

1

I'm a lucky man.

These words may seem paradoxical to anyone reading this book. To some, they may even sound like a provocation, or a challenge, but they are not meant to be. I'm in the best position to know, and if I say I'm a lucky man, it is with the absolute conviction that I've had a large share of luck in a world that is too often inhuman toward its inhabitants. But, at the same time, I must make an observation to dispel any confusion: I don't use the word "luck" in the material sense usually attributed to it. In that department, my life has dealt me more woes than blessings, as with most pencil pushers. That's fair enough, for in our line of work there are many other satisfactions. This is our compensation, and if, as you read my book, my "luck" doesn't seem self-evident, it will be because I haven't made myself clear. Another thing: this story is not a cautionary tale; it's simply my story, just as it's my luck to be a particular kind of person. This luck belongs only to me. It's my luck.

"Funny, I've got this little thing under my tongue."

That's how it all started. Twenty-odd years without seeing a doctor, an instinctive distrust of medicine and medications, and a natural optimism had given me the salutary habit of good health—a habit which is virtually an obligation for people living on the fringes of society, and grouped, for all the variety of their activities, under the somewhat pejorative rubric of "self-employed." I was one of those outcasts whom Social Security refuses to take under its wing. Independence has always been held suspect in countries with regimented freedom; it is a dangerous luxury, for it may contaminate others, and so the outcast must be made to pay for it and pay dearly. France has an instinct for conventions, as I had learned to my sorrow, and just before I discovered my "little thing," whether from laziness or perhaps a sense of premonition, I had launched on an intensive study of the literature relating to food. It was poorly paid work, to be sure, but it put me under the government's umbrella and, among other benefits, allowed me the right to be sick at someone else's expense. There are certain opportunities that mustn't be wasted.

For one month, two months, then three, life went on, and in spite of mouth washes and more drastic remedies, my "little thing," instead of getting smaller, seemed to be growing. Nobody was concerned; my "little thing" was so minor, so innocent looking, that it wasn't worth getting excited about, yet its hidden presence began to get on my nerves. I looked at it before going to sleep, it was still there when I woke up, but during the day I forgot about it. When it reached the size of a small pea, however, I decided it was overreaching itself. It gave me disagreeable ideas.

One night, I downed a drink to give me courage and

went to see a doctor who lived in the neighborhood. I had used him occasionally for my boys' childhood diseases, and knew him to be a very sensible man.

"Doctor, you don't think it's anything, do you?"

"Certainly not. Your nose and throat man will get rid of it in no time."

"But I have no nose and throat man."

"Then the simplest thing is for you to go to the hospital. I'll write a note for you."

He had trained his flashlight at length on the object of my concern, and his concluding smile was enough to bring the dead back to life: it was nothing, really nothing at all. Since I desperately wanted to share his opinion, I went home in high spirits. And the following day, I felt no apprehension at all as I sat in front of a white-coated specialist armed with a tongue depressor in one hand, a flashlight in combat position in the other.

Beforehand, I had gone through the formalities, then waited my turn, wondering what I, in such robust health, was doing among all these obviously very sick people. When my name was called out, I went into a room where patients were directed to one of the various doctors on duty sitting with their sterilized utensils in the back of little cubicles that looked like polling booths. After reading the few lines written by his colleague consigning my small growth to his care, the doctor leaned forward and examined me.

It was a long, silent examination. Then came the interrogation.

"Have you been losing weight recently?"

"No."

"Has your voice changed in any way?"

"No."

"Do you smoke?"

"A lot. Too much."

"How many cigarettes a day?"

"About thirty."

"Do you drink?"

To admit you like a drink from time to time takes a very strong character. In the confessional booth, even at the risk of blackening my soul, I would have answered yes: you don't lie to God. I may lack faith, but I do have principles. Here my answer was a little ambiguous.

"Sometimes more than I should, sometimes not at all."

So I was put down as an occasional heavy drinker, which was basically true, my life having alternated between abstinence and overindulgence, hope and depression, but I wasn't there to expand on this particular subject.

"I'm a writer," I added by way of explanation.

The cowardice of this excuse immediately struck me in all its fatuity: whether I was a writer or a plumber, what could it possibly mean to a man with few illusions about sick people's honesty? After all, it wasn't my profession that interested him. He examined me again, palpated my neck, asked me a few more questions, then suddenly stood up.

"Wait here a minute."

Why this abrupt departure? All around me, examinations were going on, people came and went, passing right by my chair. Where had my doctor gone? Some pressing need? A telephone call? He finally returned.

"Come with me. The head doctor will look at you."

It hadn't occurred to me that he had gone on my account. I was surprised, but in no way alarmed. The hospital, so often the butt of local jokes, rose in my esteem: even such an insignificant case as mine was being taken seriously. The head doctor was going to see me! Fool that I was, I almost felt flattered.

I followed the doctor into a much smaller and less animated room. Despite the many patients waiting in front of the doctor's door, he was going to see me first.

"Please sit down."

His voice was calm and steady, as were his gestures. He didn't speak as he examined me, except for an occasional yes, good, ah, yes—words with no particular significance, words that told me nothing. And any attempt to read a diagnosis on his face, expressionless by intention, would have been equally useless. All I noticed was the collar of his jacket: instead of being turned down in the usual way, it was turned up with a certain careless elegance. "The great man still has a student's dash," I said to myself. The distance between us was probably less than I had supposed.

"There is a gland there," he said to the young doctor who had remained standing beside me, then looked me squarely in the face.

"Are you free tomorrow morning?"

"Yes, Doctor."

"Good. I'll remove that little thing, and we'll do a biopsy. Come at . . ."

With an appointment for nine o'clock the following morning, I was back in the street with the disagreeable sound "biopsy" ringing in my ears. Among the medical terms that have become part of the layman's language, some have a better reputation than others; "biopsy" is frankly not good. Testing, which means the same thing, is much less offensive, and has the advantage of being less precise. I knew that my wife was sufficiently knowledgeable about medicine that the word "biopsy" would give her little pleasure. But when she suggested she go to the hospital with me, I refused point-blank. Why dramatize things?

I demoted my biopsy to the level of a casual test—just precautionary, really—and she grudgingly accepted my version. The next day, I started off again, wondering how it would all go, and imagining myself in a dentist's chair with a white towel around my neck. Instead, I found myself naked from the waist up, and strapped to an operating table. The doctor then relieved me of my "little thing."

I was home two hours later; three days later, the incision had healed and I resumed the struggle for our daily bread and my posthumous glory. It took some doing, for at the time, what with my landlord, three process servers, the tax collector, and all kinds of trouble with my work, I would gladly have dropped everything and called it quits. But that didn't occur to me. It's my luck, that luck I mentioned earlier, never to quite give up hope, no matter how low I feel. I had little time to think about my biopsy. But the day came when I had to learn the results.

It was a beautiful Thursday morning in October, and the postal workers were on strike. Contrary to what cynics may think, there was no connection between the two, but they remain inseparable in my memory. I entered the hospital in the best of spirits; I was at peace with the world and happy to be alive. The autumn sun had much to do with it, and I hoped to be done early enough to soak up a little on a park bench. I soon found my young doctor among the speleologists of nasal holes and neighboring cavities. He treated me with a detachment that augured well: the examination indicated that I was fine. As for the biopsy, he knew nothing about it, but the head doctor would give us the results in a moment. Time to smoke a couple of cigarettes on the stoop before the nurse called my name.

The head doctor greeted me with his usual courtesy, then gave me a résumé of the situation:

"You have a bad salivary gland there. We will have to get rid of it."

This didn't bother me one way or the other. One salivary gland more or less when you know that nature has given you three pairs isn't all that terrible. I said "Fine."

"All right, Doctor. How long will I be hospitalized?"

"Two weeks. Then you will have to have treatments for a while, but we'll talk about that later. When do you want to come in? It doesn't have to be tomorrow, but the sooner the better. . . ."

There were so many thing going on in my life and so many problems to solve that the time seemed poorly chosen. I would have to do this with less on my mind. Since it didn't have to be tomorrow, I said:

"How about January?"

"Ah, no. I mean much sooner than that."

Abandoning his casual manner, he got up to look at the large calendar hanging on the wall. What was the meaning of this? Was something really wrong with me? Why the hurry, why the anxiety? Still not understanding, I argued about dates, and finally, with some difficulty, I got a two-week reprieve.

"I'm counting on you, now."

"Of course."

Was there a lack of confidence? The doctor sat down again and picked up his pen.

"I'm writing a note to your dentist. I want him to remove everything metallic in your mouth."

As he was writing, I tried to collect my thoughts. He

[7]

was going to remove a gland. So why all the fuss? Maybe I was getting a little edgy?

"Take this to your dentist. Before you leave, stop by the head nurse on the floor above. She'll fill out your application. I'll draw up a sheet for her."

He started writing again, and I quickly glanced at the note he'd given me: "Dear Doctor X: The patient's surgery will include cervical neck dissection, an insertion of radium needles, and X-ray therapy. Will you please remove his dental crown and the bridgework. . . ."

I was getting the drift. So far as I was aware, radiotherapy was not used to cure a stiff neck. Everything was clear at last.

I said: "Isn't that treatment for cancer, Doctor? Do I have cancer?"

"It doesn't look good."

So far as he was concerned, the appointment was over. I didn't insist. I was no child. There are conversations that patients may desire but that doctors prefer not to prolong; it embarrasses them. Truth is not always pleasant, particularly that kind, and anyway, it was now beside the point. I had the facts.

Since I was there, I made preparations for my admission, then left the hospital as I had entered it. Not exactly the same way, though: on the surface, nothing had changed physically, but in my head, things were churning.

"I have cancer!"

I made a few tentative steps down the street. I was alone, really alone, face to face with a totally new problem: I was sick, but not just any old sickness. I had cancer. I suddenly remembered a book I had read as a child, called *Nino the Leper*. The somber story and its realistic embellishments had left a deep impression on my ten-year-old mind. Leprous, cancerous. . . . I didn't care for the similarity. But this was the wrong tack to take; I set off in another direction.

It led to a bistro. A group of postal workers were completing their appointed rounds at the bar. Most Frenchmen would be receiving no news that day, but I had news, and not of the best. In the hope of blunting the impact, I ordered a double whiskey, and as I lit a cigarette—I had no intention of giving them up—I examined my problem. Alcohol and tobacco helping, I reviewed my case with greater calm and objectivity. So I had cancer. What else is new? Did I feel any sicker now than I had two hours ago? No. Aside from one little thing under my tongue, had my health given me any trouble? Had I suffered? No. That was the good side, the positive and encouraging side. Now I had to study the ugly, bad side.

"What did he die of?" "Cancer." And people look at each other silently, giving meaningful nods of the head. "So-and-So is in very bad shape." In confidential tones, "He has cancer; he's done for." No details, the reason is understood, the verdict without appeal; everybody suppresses his fear and the family prepares the deceased for the next morning's obituaries. After a list of the dear departed's claims to glory, follows: "Died after a long illness." It doesn't fool anybody, but at least it doesn't sully his name. What bullshit!

Doing that sort of ostrich trick has never solved anything, and I've never cared for a position that makes the rear end so vulnerable. My fears quietly dissolved in scotch and smoke. There were all kinds of cancers: they came in every shape, they were treated, they were cured. Science was making progress daily. You had only to read the tabloids, even the respectable press, to find it on the front pages. Cancer sold newspapers; people in the business knew it and entertained their readers without a thought for the fact that perhaps one day they might die of the very disease that kept them fed. Nasty stuff. This curse that strikes everywhere, often without warning, or a warning that comes too late. It had come too late for my mother. What about me?

Damn it! I wasn't going to let myself be trapped by a word, for so far at least, my cancer was only a word. I couldn't let a word scare me if I was to get through this. Now I was on the right track. All I needed was to take the word, make it commonplace, roll it off the tongue like any other word. Not to fear, not to be afraid. But I was such a coward! On the other hand, perhaps people don't ask enough of themselves. . . .

"I have cancer," I repeated, and already it didn't have the same effect. It was becoming acceptable. From now on, the important thing would be the way I faced up to the disease and its consequences. I was in a position to choose my behavior, and that choice was not unimportant.

My glass was empty. The postmen had moved on from wine to stronger drink. It was almost lunchtime. Soon it would be time for me to go home; my wife and sons were waiting for me, and I would have to tell them. . . .

"Hello, Henri? It's me, Jean."

I had gotten a telephone token from the bartender and, shut up among the graffiti in the airless box, I called Henri. He is a painter, he has talent; he doesn't have any money, but he has something better to give—friendship. I knew he would understand.

"Jean, how are you?" the distant voice said in its familiar singsong. Henri is from the southwest.

"Henri, I have a question to ask you. It isn't about money. It's a serious question."

With this reassurance, I dived in.

"Henri, if you had cancer, would you tell your family?"

"Of course. Why do you ask?"

"Because I have cancer."

"Oh. . . . Where is your cancer?"

His voice didn't betray the smallest hint of surprise or concern. The news wasn't exactly welcome, but the name of the disease didn't bother him at all. I gave him a few details, and we turned to other things.

"Good-bye, Jean, old pal. I'll come see you at the hospital."

"Good-bye, Henri."

I hung up. I felt better for having told someone. It was like escaping from a kind of prison I'd almost let myself be locked up in. I paid up and, scorning the public transports, went home on foot. The sun was still warm. People sat nursing their drinks on café terraces, prolonging the waning summer; children chased each other, shouting and laughing; an old bum lay stretched out on a bench in his private nighttime, a wine bottle in an old musette bag as his pillow; a mongrel hound peed intently at the foot of a tree caged around like a bank teller. Life was beautiful. I was loving life more and more.

As I walked down the street near my home, I saw Big Joe, a local character, passing the time of day with Maurice, who owned my favorite bar and usually kept his doors wide open. They saw me and beckoned me over. I wasn't particularly thirsty but went over anyway.

After all, I had to get used to being what I was and not hide it.

"Hello, hello. What'll you have?"

"I have cancer. I'm going to be operated on in two weeks."

I had taken the second step. Joe and Maurice were not, it appeared, going to forget it lightly. Without meaning to, I had stunned two men who had seen plenty in their lives, and not just the good things: Maurice had had his leg amputated near the groin, but he clearly didn't like the idea of cancer, either. People have preferences about things like that.

A little more gently, but with the same frankness, I told my family, hoping they would be no more alarmed than I was. Amazing as it may seem, with the first shock over, I was getting used to the idea. If my disease had hit me somewhere else, if I had felt pain, I might have reacted differently, and with less surface, as well as inner, composure. Yes, I do mean inner, for I didn't see my life as threatened in any way. My cancer was no longer cancer in general, cancer whose very name instills terror: my cancer was particular, operable, and curable, since it had been caught in time and was localized. Mine was a well-bred cancer. This much said, however, I'm not totally lacking in common sense, so I told myself that even if time were of the essence, it was important not to rush into the thing headlong. The chief could be wrong; no one is infallible. And who was this doctor, anyway? I knew nothing about him. Perhaps the operation wasn't necessary. Did I really have cancer? He hadn't said it in so many words. I had a two-week reprieve, during which I must seek corroboration. Of this I had dire need. Thanks to my wife, I got it.

[12]

At my request, she made an appointment for me with a top cancer specialist, and went herself to the hospital for a copy of the results of my biopsy so that I could take it with me. The hospital turned the report over to my wife with considerable reluctance, in a sealed envelope addressed to the doctor I was going to consult. I snatched the letter from her the minute she entered the door.

"Don't you do that!" she protested. "It isn't for you."

"Sorry. I am the interested party, and I have the right to inform myself."

I read through the document without a scruple, for, although it was not addressed to me, it concerned me in a most vital way. "Anatomical and Pathological Diagnosis" was the winning heading at the top of the report. It had the smell of an autopsy. Then came the last name and first name of the patient—mine. So I was committing no indiscretion; my wife could lay her conscience to rest. "The tissue under examination involves the surface Malpighian mucous. . . ." Putting off until later the deciphering of this too hermetic text, I scanned it rapidly until I came to *"Conclusion:* Carcinoma," to which the great man had added the qualifier "epidermoid" and other epithets. In brief, I definitely had cancer. A quick look at the dictionary to make certain: cara—— carce— carci—— carcinoma: "a malignant tumor derived from epithelial tissue." There it was; I could no longer kid myself. I had cancer, all right.

I went out to have a photocopy made for my personal archives, replaced the report in an envelope, and sealed it with care. A new and official-looking envelope; the doctor would never notice.

"You've read it, of course?"

The envelope had given me away. I wasn't the first to

try the ruse. The question was more an affirmation than a question, and the young doctor sitting at his desk holding the report smiled at me. It would have been difficult to deny it without implying either that he was a fool or that I was an even bigger idiot than I in fact was.

"Obviously."

"It's easily cured, you know. Now please strip to the waist." He pointed to an examination table at the back of the room.

The ritual of examination accomplished, I put my clothes back on and we talked: the doctor who would be operating on me was a remarkable man; I couldn't be in better hands. He would report to him and see me after I left the hospital. If it proved necessary, he would give me some additional treatment. Nothing to worry about. . . .

"Doctor, do I need to take any precautions at home?"

"What do you mean by precautions?"

"I don't know . . . hygienic precautions. . . . Am I contagious?"

The memory of *Nino the Leper* was hard to shake off, and my knowledge of cancer was no better than the next man's. It was a question I'd been pondering, and I didn't want to put it into words in front of my wife. I can take the bad news better alone, God knows. It was one of the reasons I didn't want her here for the interview. Also, I was afraid her presence would blunt our frankness. Had she come with me, the doctor might have tried to spare me, then later, unbeknownst to me, he would tell her the truth, which she would do everything to keep from me—all exactly what I wanted to avoid. As for my being contagious, he was categorical: there was absolutely nothing to fear. Nino the Leper could put his clothes back on with a clear conscience.

"Try to cut down on the smoking," he said as he saw me to the door.

"I'll try, Doctor."

He knew perfectly well I was lying, and so did I, of course. Still and all, I thought it was better to seem conciliatory toward a man in whom I was placing so much faith.

As I puffed on the cigarette I so badly needed, I began to think about this "faith" that was trying to work its way into my intentions. It was not without an element of danger; on many an occasion, life had made me pay dearly for my unwarranted faith, and had left me none the wiser. This time, I wasn't going to make that mistake. It was a matter of my health, and I had a soft spot for this bag of bones I'd been dragging around all these years. I must stop being gullible and leave nothing to chance.

The next few days weren't very pleasant for me. I was torn between asking for advice from my wife, friends, and relatives—wouldn't their affection help set me on the right track? Isn't it a known fact that people are wiser about other people than they are about themselves?—and following the instinct for self-preservation that warned me to keep them at bay. I gave in to the former, and for the next few days, I was subjected to massive doses of goodwill, most of it contradictory. So-an-So's father was treated by such-and-such a doctor for fifteen years with no operation and was still in the best of health. A friend's aunt whom we thought done for found this remarkable surgeon—I must go see him. The son of a cousin's aunt, given up by everybody, was now in enviable health.

Everybody had a cancer cure, a name, an address, a new and revolutionary therapy to recommend. Miracle remedies, tomorrow's and even the day after tomorrow's, from the waters of Lourdes to donkey's urine, from the summits of medicine to pure quackery. All my nearest and dearest were armed to fight my cancer. They meant well, they wanted me well, only I hadn't forgotten that I had once been in their shoes and thought I was doing the right thing by telling someone that "Doctor X" would make his cancer disappear with injections and magic nostrums. I was listened to, and I regret it. That someone was a close relative for whom I felt a deep affection: he spent a great deal of money for nothing. Perhaps where classic medicine is still powerless, faith is the court of last resort.

My friend Henri's wife finally managed to break down my resistance. Having been operated on for almost total deafness by a renowned specialist, she persuaded me, against my wife's better judgment, to go with her to seek her doctor's advice.

The waiting room at the clinic had deep comfortable chairs in contrast to the barren discomfort of the hospital's. There was no comparison between this modern building and the decrepit pile, soon to be demolished, in which I was to have my operation. Wouldn't I be better off here? Hadn't I been rushing things a bit? What if this new doctor found surgery uncalled for? Was his competence greater than my doctor's? If they disagreed, I would have to choose, or consult a third man, and why not a fourth . . . ?

"I am about to make a terrible mistake!" As the minutes rolled by, the conviction grew that I could avoid it if I moved in time. I had no personal appointment with the doctor; my friend was only going to mention me during the course of her periodic examination. My departure wouldn't phase him in the slightest; he didn't know I was there, that I even existed. In the next minute, the door would open. . . . Complaining that I'd been kept waiting too long, that I had another important appointment, I thanked the surprised nurse, mumbled a few hurried excuses to my friend, and bolted. Once outside, I had the sensation of having just escaped a great danger.

As time passed, I realized I hadn't been such an idiot. If this specialist had given me the same advice as the chief at the hospital, it would have changed nothing; if it had been different, things would have been hellishly complicated, opening up a future of endless comparison-shopping, of "if I had only knowns," and "perhaps I should haves," and all the litany of useless regrets that eat up people's lives more surely even than cancer. From then on, I embarked on the only possible path, the right path, because I had the best doctors, and I would be operated on and cured under the best possible conditions. The Coué method had much to recommend it: every day in every way I would get better and better. I would put my complete faith in those in charge of my health. My decision was final, the choice made. I was pleased and not a little proud of myself; I alone had determined my fate—or at least, my cancer's fate. After all, it and I must keep our distance.

I have the best doctors in Paris . . . the best qualified . . . the most capable . . . the most. . . .

With this affirmation, I would devise a shield and forge an armor that must be impervious to all doubts, whatever their source. I would be invulnerable to doubt; I had passed the point of no return. This much was settled. Now I had to deal with my financial situation, which seemed much thornier than the state of my health. My hospital stay posed burning questions about my solvency. My brother, with his usual kindness, moved into the breach.

"Your health comes first. . . . How much do you need?" My brother doesn't waste words. Once again, he was throwing me and mine a life preserver.

With this worry behind me, I had the peace of mind necessary to prepare for my stay at the hospital; I could now view it as an adventure, or better still, as an interesting and not particularly frightening experience. These days, who hasn't had an operation? Hadn't I already had one? Why, everybody has operations, it's perfectly normal. . . . Yes, but not for what ailed me. I could tell just from watching people's reactions when I mentioned it: they were already buying a funeral wreath. . . .

If I had decided to bare my soul, it was not for the pleasure of the thing. It was simply that by not hiding the truth I was helping myself; I was facing up to the disease. I was showing courage, and in the process of showing courage, I became courageous.

In offices, with storekeepers, with my friends, in bistros, wherever my steps led me, I would say, if the occasion presented itself: "By the way, I'm going to be operated on next week."

"You are? What for?"

"Oh, cancer."

It had a chilling effect. I had tamed the word with such success that I used it with almost insulting casualness. I was defying the accepted wisdom. There was often a look of reproach on their faces. But my intentions were the best. People speak freely about cars, don't they? As modern plagues go, cars seemed to be doing very well. But cancer was different; when you speak of cancer, you imply suffering. And since I looked plump and healthy, my news inspired disbelief.

"You have cancer? Don't make me laugh!"

"It's God's truth. I'm not joking."

Sometimes I was almost driven to show them the photocopy of my biopsy report to prove it. But I refrained because explaining my carcinoma was too complicated. Cancer they knew about; carcinoma, no. Besides, everybody knew me to be a man who likes a good laugh; coming from a writer, a creator of fantasies, anything was possible. I was furious at the idea that people could think me guilty of such bad taste when I was only trying to be honest. No, I wasn't joking, no, it was no laughing matter; cancer was a disease like any other, easily treated and cured. I don't know that I convinced anybody, but on the other hand, I was increasingly certain that what I was saying was true. I have a fertile imagination.

In keeping with the crusade I was preaching—chiefly for my own benefit—I simplified the problem further by demoting my cancer to the level of an only slightly malignant tumor. I conceded that the disease did come in less attractive forms and that I could have decided against the operation, but, I insisted, in the great majority of cases, there was a chance, if not of total cure, of a remission lasting many years. Sometimes I ran smack into a stone wall:

"If I had cancer, I'd shoot myself."

"You'd be a damn fool," I'd answer coolly. "The idea has never entered my head."

The days trickled by. One November morning, I said good-bye to my neighborhood and entered the hospital. I was more curious than worried. Along with the word, I'd tamed the thing itself.

My wife, who had done her best to hide her anxiety, accompanied me. She critically examined the ward, one of whose eight beds was reserved for me. Nothing is ever good enough for those who love you: I must have this, I lacked that; she would be back in the afternoon with what was obviously wanting. That's the way women are. I thought everything was fine. I needed nothing except the two crowns and the bridge my dentist had removed the day before as he bemoaned the fact that he had been forced to destroy such beautiful handiwork. This was especially noble of him, since another dentist had done it. The thought that in the not too distant future I might consign the restoration work to him probably consoled him. He felt obliged to tell me the number of patients he had who had undergone the same operation and were still in excellent health. The warmth of his farewell was tinged with a quite understandable hope that he would be seeing me again.

With my few possessions stashed away in the bedside table and myself decked out in pale blue pajamas, my wife reluctantly left me, after a shower of kisses and a welter of advice. I watched her walk down the center aisle of the ward, reach the door, turn to give me a last smile, and disappear. . . . Then, a feeling of relief came over me such as I hadn't felt in years. The last tie that bound me to my daily life was ruptured. All my worries had been left at the hospital door—process servers, creditors, and all my other bugaboos. The hell with my worries; I was protected, beyond their reach. Anyone who hasn't experienced that feeling has missed one of the most precious varieties of pleasure. I was the exhausted traveler who has finally reached his goal, the spent mountain climber resting in the shelter, the harried medieval vagrant finding asylum in a church. The right of asylum! What a noble invention that is! That is what Social Security had granted me. I was a privileged person.

I lit a cigarette and, while pretending to read one of the books I'd brought along, I sneaked a look at the small universe in which I now found myself. Boarding school, military service, and prison camp had prepared me for these first contacts which so often determine the future of one's communal life, although this one was to be short-lived. Patients come and go. In this respect, a hospital ward is like a train compartment: people get off, others get on, the train starts up again, you strike up new acquaintances, make conversation, share a stretch of the trip. Then the train stops, the cell as previously constituted loses one element, sometimes two, takes on replacements, and everything begins all over again. Some are on long trips, others on shorter. My ticket was for two weeks; I wasn't going far.

As was proper, I made the first move. A word here, a cigarette offered there, a newspaper loaned, information sought, and in a few minutes I had been adopted by my new family and initiated into the customs of the place. Our ward had no one with major surgery: one man had broken his jaw in a car accident, another had a deviated septum; there was a tonsillectomy, a skin graft, a man from Martinique awaiting some form of extraction, two other odd jobs, and me. Apart from the tonsillectomy who was still in pain, everyone else was in good health and had nothing on his mind but to have as good a time as possible. It was a propitious beginning; I felt as if I were on holiday. I made no mystery of why I was there but made so little of it that nobody took a grim view of my case.

The only exception was the nurse who came in early the next morning:

"I have to get a blood sample. Come with me, please."

"Certainly."

"What are you here for?"

"Cancer."

"What!"

I had never seen a look of such stupor on a face. The young woman was literally struck dumb, so politeness dictated that I come to her rescue.

"I have a carcinoma in a sublingual gland," I said with an ingratiating smile.

"And you know it?" she asked, still doubtful.

"Of course. It's in my report. Want to see it?"

She gave me a thin smile. "Well, you certainly sound pleased with yourself."

Pleased with myself? What did she mean by that? I followed her into the treatment room where she had to try several times before she could get her needle into my vein. Perhaps she was still too wrought up. Once she had the amount of blood needed for the tests indicated, I was taken in tow by an orderly with a Mediterranean accent.

"Get your dressing gown. We're going for a walk. It's better to get everything over with today because tomorrow is Saturday and everybody's off."

"What about Sunday?"

"Sunday too."

As we went from one section to another, from X rays to electrocardiograms, I chatted with my companion. He had been working here a long time; he liked the place and planned to stay until he was ready to retire to his native Corsica.

"You'll like it here, you wait and see. It may be old, but it's small. The patient isn't lost here like in those huge modern factories with the endless corridors."

His sweeping gesture suggested the vastness of modern buildings and it conveyed the contempt that the owner of a jalopy feels for a Cadillac he can't afford. I agreed with him wholeheartedly. Perhaps wrongly, I know, but I too was put off by those enormous assembly lines for the sick, put off by their functional perfection, put off by everything anonymous and egalitarian, put off by the thought that I would become just another perforated card. I was too old to change. I wanted to live and die with my personality intact. I did not impart my opinion to my philosophical friend, but I was certain that by the time I returned to my ward, he would have me classified.

"There are good patients and bad, like in everything else. Some patients are never happy; they complain about the food, the staff, the doctors, everything. They're not happy here, and there's nothing we can do about it. Nothing's perfect, that's for sure; people with any sense know that."

As he left he said casually, "When I have time, I'll bring you a spittoon. You can use it as an ashtray." He had given me top classification! . . .

I have no intention of giving a detailed account of my stay in the hospital or of praising the arrangements. It was no Club Méditerranée, but the five days I spent there left me with only pleasant memories. Once in hospital pajamas, stripped of the outer signs, the trappings of pride and individuality, men readily pick up the elementary and long-forgotten instinct for fraternity. In many respects, it's a childish fraternity, but a touching one. Cared for, fed, watched over, by turns encouraged or scolded, pampered or threatened by all levels of the white-clad staff, adults and even the very old go back to what, in their heart of hearts, they've never stopped being: children. I liked this return to "kindergarten." I didn't read a single page; I had no wish to, and actually, I had no time.

Between the visitors that brought us the distant echoes of the world outside, we concentrated on the closed circuit of our cruise ship. We were not allowed to leave the ward without being accompanied. To stretch our legs, we could go as far as the stairs and visit with the occupants of other wards; only one corridor was out of bounds.

"The people in there are in bad shape," one of my companions told me in a conspiratorial tone.

"In bad shape." It didn't take me long to guess why. There was cancer in there. I christened it the "elephant wing" because the patients in that ward had long tubes coming out of their noses. They couldn't speak because of the tubes, and they came to cast cheerless eyes at the television set in our room.

I wondered about the function of those tubes. It went out of the nose and up, and was held in that position by a gauze band wrapped around the head like a halo. Out of tact, and to avoid revealing my ignorance, I refrained from asking the reason for this nasal extension. It obviously had a depressing effect on its wearers, for these people seemed weighted down with a haunting gloom which the trunk alone did not explain. I decided not to dwell on it any longer; it might jeopardize the peaceful rhythm of my days and the tranquillity of my nights. You learn to be very self-centered in a hospital.

My operation was looming. Sunday morning, I decided to go to mass. As I've said, I have no religious faith, but that doesn't prevent me from wishing I had and envying those who have experienced its blessings. So it seemed perfectly natural to make a gesture that couldn't possibly displease the Lord who I hoped existed even though He had brought me no convincing proof. In my particular circumstances, to resort to divine protection seemed the most elementary kind of precaution. Besides, I was making an effort that might win me some points. Ever since the church had turned demagogic by offering a supermarket religion abetted by a self-service communion, I had felt less guilty about not taking part in the Sunday ritual I'd cast off in my youth. I may be poor, but I want no part of a mystery at reduced prices; the one I seek cannot be marked down.

To my pious and worthy project I rallied the man from Martinique, who was a practicing Catholic, and Aldo, the man with the skin graft, who was not, but saw in the outing a chance for a change of air. I had to bargain long and hard with the head nurse and vouch for our good conduct before I got her authorization. In most women's minds, the hour for mass implies a visit to the nearest bistro, and the nurses knew that leaving the hospital, even in regulation pajamas and dressing gowns, was no handicap to a patient determined to have a drink. That was not our idea, and my intentions, though not entirely disinterested, had a higher aim: I wanted to improve my odds in exchange for a small sacrifice. Surely this was no sin. Once again, I was wrong.

We had just sat down on the empty benches in the silent chapel when the padre came charging out of the sacristy and stood before us breathing fire:

"What are you doing here?"

In such a place and on a Sunday morning, the question seemed odd, even unsuitable, but as I was responsible for our trio, it behooved me to answer politely:

"We've come for mass," I said as humbly as possible.

"That's right, Father," the man from Martinique chimed in. "We were saying a few prayers while waiting."

"There is no mass for patients."

And he explained bluntly that morning mass was only

for those giving blood, so we had no right to be there. We could attend mass in the afternoon, but now we were not welcome. Looking more like a prosecutor than a priest as he stood, arms crossed, at the foot of the altar, he bade us leave and watched until we were gone. The knowledge that the blood I might well be needing would come from a Christian in a full state of grace did not make up for the fact that we were being thrown out of the house of the Lord. Our expulsion didn't seem very Christian, and I was annoyed for having led my companions into such a misadventure. Aldo took it especially hard.

"For Christ's sake!" he said, glaring at the closed door. "The one time I set foot in church, they kick me out. The bastard treated us as if we were unclean!"

The West Indian accepted our fate in silence, with the stoicism of the true believer. If he felt any indignation, it was tempered by his respect for religion and its servants. God's ways are sometimes mysterious; perhaps the priest had misinterpreted orders from on high. Caught between Aldo's irritation and the indulgent passivity of the man from Martinique, I took the ambiguous stance of the coward: I wavered. I don't like to judge what I don't understand, and any intransigence on my part could threaten what I hoped to gain by my good intentions. Prudence, prudence.

Like landlords inspecting their domains, we made an unhurried tour of the hospital. Everything was calm, peaceful, bathed in happy torpor. It was clear that dying in a hospital on Sunday morning wasn't done. You disappear, you are extinguished, you enter into the peace of the Lord if you so choose, but you don't die the same way as on other days.

The three of us decided not to breathe a word about the little incident. Our silence would protect our ambiguous beliefs: we were Catholics, not just poor bastards unworthy of taking part in a mass. So we returned with no need to explain anything, and with the happy faces of men who have done their duty.

With a better dinner, and more and longer visits, Sunday ran its smooth course and would have ended thus had not a piece of news raced from ward to ward, finally reaching ours. It appeared that the priest had surprised some patients breaking into the chapel collection box that morning, but the culprits had escaped. There were three of them. The number was too precise to leave any doubts in our minds. So I took it upon myself to explain everything. My character may have its weak points, but I had not come to the hospital with the intention of making off with the church offering, aided and abetted by two accomplices recruited on the premises. It would have made far more sense to tackle the hospital safe. . . . The evidence was in our favor, but we weren't completely absolved until the penitent and very annoyed priest appeared on the scene. Still upset by a theft committed the night before and taking off from there on the debatable principle that the guilty always return to the scene of the crime, the sight of us in the chapel had brought on his unfortunate reaction. To admit one's mistakes is a virtue given to few. After consulting my acolytes, I granted him absolution without going into the Hail Marys and Lord's Prayer he would have exacted from us had it been the other way around. It wasn't in my line of work, and I didn't know the litany called for. Too strong a dose and I might have offended the saintly man. I must have struck the right tone, for, on leaving, he promised to pray for us. I couldn't have hoped for more.

If I have dwelt too long on this incident of the collection box, it's because it was the only thing that in any way troubled the surprising euphoria I had been feeling ever since I entered the hospital. As with happiness in general, it can't be described. Happiness is too relative and too individual to be understood by others, but in the five days of hospital routine, I had put on pounds of well-being. It was balm to the soul. To say that I never thought about my coming operation would be a lie. I thought of it with intense apprehension, so I tried to push it out of my thoughts as much as possible.

My only other setback came when I ran into an orderly from surgery pushing his wagon on which a patient lay, wrapped in a blanket.

"Your turn soon!" he said merrily, indifferent to the appearance of his passenger, who looked far from jaunty. The wagon pusher was always as gay as his patient was pale and torpid—a mummy sprouting all manner of tubes. Of all those tubes, there was that one that really bothered me: the one that came from some unknown depths and exited through a nostril, turning the mummy into an elephant. Cancer and this tube seemed to go together. Since I had the former, would I automatically be endowed with the latter? The luck of being unusually stupid about all medical matters had made it possible for me to accept cancer, and to make mine completely different from all others. My cancer was unique; it was in my image.

It's very important to have such convictions. That is why I had a very vague hope that I wouldn't become an elephant. Alcohol and tobacco: I had all the necessary certificates to make me an elephant, but still I fought it off. Uncertainty is the most uncomfortable of all sensations, and I was determined to resolve it somehow.

Patients tend to view their doctors as belonging to a superior and distant world to which they have no access.

It is the fearsome world of diagnosis and scalpel, the mysterious world of experts from whom miraculous cures are expected. Doctors know this, and from the lowliest medical student to the greatest surgeon, a hermetic posture, serious or smiling according to the individual temperament, is the golden rule of the profession. With their inscrutable faces and private jargon, they build a wall of lies between the patient and his disease that is impervious to everything but hope. Perhaps they are right—in general.

As a beginning patient, determined to be one only temporarily and in moderation, I was naive enough to accept the doctors' words. I know now they weren't Holy Scripture, but that in no way diminishes my confidence in the men who have been treating me all these years with devotion and skill. I'm sure they don't tell me the whole truth. They'll lie to me tomorrow if they decide it's in my best interests, and for that I thank them.

For fear of looking ridiculous, I didn't want to bring up the business of the wretched tube in front of witnesses. Trying to corner a doctor when he wasn't making his brief morning visit or striding down the corridor with his train of followers wasn't easy. I still hadn't succeeded when Tuesday came and I was taken from my small and cherished community to the elephants' quarters. I was put in a double room, one bed already occupied by a patient who looked very poorly and—bad omen—had a trunk directed straight up at the ceiling.

Early the next morning, I was awaiting the hour of truth with a great show of indifference that fooled nobody, and smoking one cigarette after another to calm my nerves, when I saw my doctor hurrying down the hall. I just had time to stop him in midflight.

"Doctor"—I had carefully prepared my strategy—"if

during my operation, you should discover something more serious than you expect, please don't tell my wife."

It got me the response it deserved.

"Oh, there's nothing to worry about. I know what I'm going to find."

The doctor was already off and running, and I had to pursue him to get to the heart of the matter.

"Am I going to have a tube in my nose?"

He looked at me briefly, his eyes filled with wonder.

"A tube? Whatever for? As I told you, you'll have a radium needle for six days. . . . See you soon."

No time to ask him more; he was already rushing down the stairs four at a time. Great doctors are often in a hurry.

Suddenly, along came the cheery wagon pusher, and he invited me aboard his vehicle. Chatting away, he wrapped me up in a blanket. Down an asthmatic elevator, into the operating room, then onto the table to the accompaniment of casual banter from the professional entourage.

Up to then, everything had seemed to go very well. But inside my head, a horror movie started up in which I was the leading actor, playing an innocent victim. The horror deepened when, my feet and wrists bound and helpless, I found myself alone, my eyes fixed on the operating room light that, even unlit, left me with no illusions: my future was inescapable.

Memories, worries, thoughts, hopes, everything in my brain whirled and tumbled. I had given my life over to others, and I could do nothing but try to pray. People were moving silently around me making preparations and the movie of my terror kept unwinding when suddenly the most unexpected thing happened: a hand took hold of mine and stroked it. I couldn't see who it belonged to, but from the softness of the hand and the comfort I took from the contact, I guessed it must be a woman's. My fingers interlaced with hers, responded to her pressure, and everything inside me grew calm. A woman's hand, nothing more than a woman's hand. My gratitude was indescribable.

I felt less gratitude for the hand that slapped me awake. I have a very disagreeable memory of that awakening: the painful sensation of suffocating. And for good reason: I didn't have one tube in my nose, I had two. They were being too generous! One nostril was unblocked, I began to breathe, and my spirits picked up. It was then that I made the humiliating discovery that I was indeed an elephant like all the others and that the doctor had lied to me.

Once I was fully conscious of the uninviting spectacle I presented, I asked my wife in writing (for I couldn't speak) to let no one besides her, least of all my boys, come to visit me. I didn't want anyone to see me thus violated. It was a matter of pride, to be sure, but also the fear of inspiring pity. I am capable of pity and can feel compassion for human misery, but that I should inspire pity seemed to me an intolerable fall from grace. Anything, dear God, but pity!

During breakfast the morning after my operation, my mind more or less lucid though my legs wobbly, I learned from my neighbor the reason for my detestable tube and the way to use it. It was very simple. You introduced a funnel into the end and, holding it with one hand, poured your pot of liquid nourishment into it with the other. The expression "to have a snootful" came to mind. Direct from the orifice to stomach; just like a car at a gas pump, I was "filling her up."

Its alimentary function finished, I hooked the trunk smartly to my forehead. What I must look like! I picked up a mirror: bandages, adhesive tape, tube, and a missing tooth somehow lost in the fray, did little for my appearance. I may be no Greek god, but up to then, I had liked myself well enough. Now, viewed with all possible indulgence, I was not an attractive sight.

At that moment doubts began to creep in surreptitiously: before, to all intents and purposes, I had been in the best of health; now, I was sick. Had I been right to have this operation? Now I realized what made my other tubed friends look so sad. Wounded in their flesh, isolated in their silence, they too must be asking themselves over and over again, "Was I right to have this operation?" without being able to find a comforting answer. I realized that, for all my effort, I had not been able to escape the moral anguish of that question. It took me forty-eight hours to come to the sensible conclusion that, whether I regretted it or not, what was done was done, irrevocably done, and there was nothing I could do to change it.

To reaffirm my faith in my doctors became an indispensable necessity for my moral and physical health. I had acted well; it had been in my best interests to have the operation. To reinforce my conviction, I even condoned the doctor's lie: he had guessed that I dreaded the tube, but he was the boss.

Six days. The Six Day Bicycle Race, the Six Day War. Six days can be short; they can be very long. My six days weren't short, but they did finally come to an end, and, as my surgeon promised, the radium needle was removed, along with my trunk.

"Try a shave now," was all he said on his next visit. He spoke little, but always to the point. A shave was indeed indicated.

I resumed my place among my fellowman, my optimism intact, but not my neck, at least on the left side. To judge from the number of clamps, they had done a thorough job. I could once again talk, laugh, be myself. Out of consideration for my roommate, I moderated my joy. A much younger man than I, he had for weeks, and probably would far into the future, stoically endured something far worse than what I'd endured poorly for a few days. In spite of everything he had gone through, he still didn't know he had cancer, and his wife, who came to see him every day, had decided it was better not to tell him.

I wouldn't have liked that. To leave to others the burden of carrying the full weight of one's illness without taking one's own share, to force those you love to go on playing this harrowing game seemed to me totally dishonest. Any arguments to the contrary were highly debatable. A conspiracy of silence, or the truth? I think with horror on the life I would have imposed on my family if they had felt obliged to lie to me constantly to keep me from hearing the word "cancer." What luck that I had been the first to know!

Actually, though, my wife knew before I did. Women are clever devils. She had gone to see the doctor the day before I was to find out the results of my biopsy. He had made no attempt to conceal his pessimistic prognosis. He was almost certain I had cancer even before seeing the lab report. Dreading my displeasure at this chicanery, and there she wasn't wrong, she only admitted it to me much later. It also explained why the doctor was on his guard with me.

She must have painted a vivid picture of my questionable character, with the best intentions, naturally. At least she was now delivered of her useless secret which she would have found very hard to carry.

My nose unstoppered, vocal chords freed, tongue

ready for conversation, and with an impressive scar that wanted showing off, I held court, making the most of the role of recent surgical victim who scoffs at his small miseries. I have to admit that it took some effort, but I was a good actor. Relatives, friends, all the visitors in my narrow "alley"—the restricted space around my bed—congratulated me on my bravery. Anybody can do it if he has the wit to call on his willpower. Willpower is a quality often underused, as I am the first to admit.

Little by little, I discovered my willpower. I was less confident when it came to facing the prospect of giving up smoking. I had picked up the habit very young, and as the years went by, it had become more essential to me than food or drink. The doctors didn't actually forbid me to smoke; they simply advised against it. Deprived of tobacco for almost a week, my throat still sore from the tube, this appeared to be the unhoped-for opportunity to break off my long servitude. As if waiting to entrap me, my cigarettes and lighter lay on my bedside table. During that first day I was tempted many times, but, distracted by visits and the hospital routine, I had not yet succumbed. By evening, however, the need became intolerable.

"If I take one, just one, it's all over," I said, feeling the pack but hesitating to pick it up. A visit from my brother-in-law did the trick.

"Watch me," I said, lighting a cigarette. "Watch me closely."

He looked confused.

"You are watching me do something for the last time." I inhaled deeply, gave my lungs the benefit of a long treat, and slowly exhaled. Then, ceremoniously, I crushed the cigarette in my spittoon-ashtray.

"See. It's over. I will never smoke again."

And I have never smoked since that day.

What pride I have today is based on that victory. I thought I didn't have the willpower. When I state that to stop smoking was the hardest thing I've ever done, I am speaking the truth. I could have made the resolution alone, but, knowing how weak I was, I wasn't likely to keep it long. Having a witness made all the difference. I challenged myself by throwing an extra trump on the trick: my pride. You don't have to be Oriental to dislike "losing face." 1906115

I have kept my word, and repentant smokers know the price you pay when you break this most ordinary and agreeable of habits. All the stratagems I resorted to, all the varieties of candies I sucked to outwit the craving, would have been useless but for the intensity of my vigilance. One moment's relaxation, one second's weakness, and I would have had to begin all over again.

I can't count the number of nights I have dreamed I was caressing a pretty girl—dreams, after all, are the legal tender of faithful husbands. But I still wake up with a guilty start if I dream I've been smoking. Now I usually carry cigarettes with me so that I can offer them to others with the satisfaction of knowing I don't smoke myself. If I sometimes make too much of my abstinence, I hope I'll be forgiven. I don't mean to show off or make others feel guilty. It's simply my reward for good behavior.

The clamps were removed two days after the tube, and I was able to appreciate the aesthetic changes wrought on my natural proportions. The left side of my jaw seemed to protrude alarmingly over a diminished neck, giving me a Modigliani-like profile. Now, Modigliani may be a great painter, but I didn't like the havoc wreaked on my face. As an old soldier in an earlier and more successful war than this one, I christened the furrow which my razor worked with delicate precaution, "the bayonet trench." Memories pop up at odd times: when I was ten, I visited the battlefields at Verdun, which will never be done digesting their dead, and the sight of all those bayonets still sticking out of the soil left a lasting impression. Each steel point represented the extension of a rifle buried with the man grasping it as he had been about to go over the top. A bombardment had decided otherwise. Fifty-seven lives stopped at the selfsame moment. Even if we do these things more efficiently now, it will always be those dead who symbolize for me the horror and waste of war.

The next day, the doctor announced that everything was going so well that there was no reason for me to stay on in the hospital.

"What about the radiotherapy?" I asked, like a poor fool demanding his rights who, since he is paying nothing, is afraid he won't get his due.

"You don't need it. Rest up and come see me in a month."

I thanked him somewhat ungraciously, said good-bye left and right, and the next day I was back in circulation. I returned home less frisky than I had left, holding on to my wife's arm, quite oblivious to the fact that she was barely able to hold me up. The affection lavished on a person who has been through even a short illness prods him irresistibly toward an appalling egotism. Having been catalogued and computerized, the patient at first accepts coddling with gratitude, then comes to expect it, and even exaggerates things to make his case more dramatic.

I was no exception, and I might have slid into a spoiled and protracted convalescence if I hadn't been abruptly called back to reality. One morning, my wife fainted in the street. And little more than a week after my return home, she was in the hospital, fearing—although she would not admit it—what I feared even more. One cancer in a family was enough; two seemed excessive. As she had for me, I talked to the specialist who examined her. He reassured me that my wife was only suffering from an ulcer, probably brought on by concern over my illness. I had had two weeks in the hospital; she had two weeks. We got equal time, as it were, and life picked up where it left off.

Well, not exactly. My worries hadn't gone away during my absence. They were the same as when I had checked them at the hospital door. I hadn't died, so I had gained only a respite. It had now run out. The work in progress, projects, tentative starts, nothing was changed, everything was only waiting to begin again.

Yes, there was one small change, a detail that may seem of no importance: I couldn't wear a tie. It was a question of symmetry. My neck, that is, my neck in its new form, made the problem insoluble. The undamaged neck of a strong young man, an intact neck, is a thing of beauty. Mine wasn't. And since it looked even worse with a tie, I had to find some way to hide it until it came to terms with itself.

So I adopted an ascot. In this carnival period we're living in, where people's clothes come from attic trunks or the neighborhood thrift shop (and in hope of achieving distinction, everybody ends up looking the same), my ascots seemed to me a blameless frippery. I might even look like a decadent artist or a dashing movie producer.

My hopes weren't disappointed. One day, as I was

crossing the street dutifully between the lines, I was almost struck down by a car. As the driver jammed on the
brakes, he yelled out: "Why don't you look where you're
going, you fag!" I smiled and said nothing. Some insults
have the effect of a compliment. I like my ascot, and
women, too much to have felt insulted.

2

With my work at home, visits to various offices, meetings with friends, stops at bistros to chat and linger over a soft drink, I was sucked back into the familiar routine, explaining when necessary, and even when it wasn't, that my absence had been due to an operation for cancer. Time passed. Except for the monthly checkups at the hospital and the even rarer visits to the doctor who was watching over my general health, I would have forgotten all about my cancer. My illness no longer had top priority. If I happened to mention it during the course of a conversation, it was with growing detachment and even some humor. I'm a bit of a ham; all writers are, especially the second-raters, which does not necessarily mean the lesser known.

Giving up tobacco and the substitution of candy soon had their effect. As a middle-class Frenchman, sedentary out of professional necessity and resistant to the benefits of physical culture indoors or out, I started to get fat. I made a few timid efforts, like taking walks and halfhearted attempts at dieting. But like most men, I considered a little fat a sign of well-being and felt that I deserved envy rather than pity.

Some, seeing me look so well, questioned my doctors' wisdom. They weren't stupid or ignorant, but cultivated, intelligent people who considered themselves knowledgeable about many things, including medicine. The first to do it was a man for whom I felt great affection and who I knew felt the same way about me. He did it in the presence of my wife, which didn't help matters. For her sake, I tried to steer the conversation to other subjects, but when my friend had left, the thing I dreaded most happened.

"You heard what he said. Perhaps you shouldn't have . . ." I didn't let her finish the sentence, but broke in sharply: "Oh, no. Not from you! I don't give a damn if he or other people say it, but not you. I did what I had to do, and let's not go over it again. Anybody who thinks otherwise can go to hell."

There are always more than enough reasons for starting a family quarrel; no need to think up new ones. Her temperament is different from mine, which is unfortunate, but I do understand what she goes through. When our roles were being assigned, I was favored: I got the easy one, and it isn't altogether fair.

The warm weather was around the corner. Spring, in a city like Paris, with an ascot around your neck, presents problems I hadn't foreseen. An ascot of even the lightest fabric makes you very hot. But I couldn't see doing without it. My wife kept saying: "You exaggerate. It barely shows."

I'm not blind, and mirrors don't lie. Whether I was less handsome or more unattractive—take your pick—concerned me little. You deteriorate with time, as does a house, so whether it's sooner or later makes little difference. When I see some poor soul, man or woman, whom fate has dealt an ugly face, and then realize that that person has had to live with it all his life, make love with it, cry with it, it's brought home to me again how lucky I am. But to inflict my scar on friends or strangers just because there are still uglier sights in the world—no!

You remember a scar, it registers on the memory. I wanted to be remembered for other things. It wasn't pride, it was plain ordinary decency. I had spent too much time looking around hospital waiting rooms not to be aware of it. My scar wasn't particularly repellent, it was even what surgeons call a "good-looking" scar. But there is an enormous difference between letting it be seen and showing it off, which has to do with respect for others as well as for oneself. So I went on sweating in my ascot.

Finally the day came when I was able to leave the hot and humid city and smell the fresh salt air of my native province. The news of my operation had preceded me long before, and as it traveled by word-of-mouth, it had become somewhat deformed. Only the essential facts remained. An old and outspoken friend not overburdened with tact was the first to set me straight:

"Well, how are you? I heard you were dead!"

"As you see, I'm not."

Of course he saw it, since I was standing there in front of him, shaking his hand. But in his eyes I saw some confusion. He went on:

"Didn't you have something this past winter?"

"Yes, I had cancer."

"Ah, that's right. Somebody told me."

Reassured, he broke into a wide smile.

"You've put on weight, though. But you're okay for now?"

My burial was only deferred. Many a family must

have thought I was risen from the dead. In the provinces, even more than in Paris, cancer is considered a fatal disease, and when it's a question of putting somebody under the sod, they're always impatient. If necessary, they will even pick up a shovel and help dig the hole.

Whether they had thought me dead or alive was immaterial. The weather was beautiful, and I was happy to be among the living. I picked up with old friends, some of whom lived there all year, others who came from far away, all of them eager for these annual summer reunions. One of those particularly dear to me gave my profile an expert's appraisal.

"If you ask me, I like you better from that side. While they were at it, why didn't they make the two sides the same?"

There's a real friend for you.

I was working harder than usual during the holidays. I had a television drama contracted for two years earlier that was due for production, as well as some other ideas I'd proposed, and, in the hope of being liberated from my assembly-line labors, I was finishing off an admittedly commercial comedy. I didn't know the ORTF (the French state-owned television company) very well at the time, and the theater not at all. But I didn't think it made any difference. My optimism never falters. . . .

I was no less optimistic when, on my return to Paris, I had to go before the Magistrate's Court and explain why I hadn't paid my premium into the Pension Fund, an abusive and tenacious fund well known to authors. With great politeness I asked the judge: "Do you think it makes sense to spend money on an eventual retirement when you've just been operated on for cancer?"

Some arguments carry weight, and I was granted an

exemption. But the law was not discouraged by this temporary setback: I had to do battle every year, and each time come forth with new doctors' certificates. Had I needed a reason for hope, their determination provided it. Whether or not I had cancer, they were bent on providing for my retirement. I found this encouraging, especially since I was eager to go on living, if alert and lucid, to a very ripe old age. On the other hand, it seemed to me absurd that I should save for later the money I so desperately needed now. Besides, retirement for a writer, painter, or anyone whose life is spent creating something, is a meaningless word.

One visit a month the first year, one every other month the second, one every three months the next: at this decelerated rate, my visits to the hospital were becoming a routine formality. I met with the staff, gossiped with the nurses when they had the time (which was rare), joked with the orderlies on duty, asked about those who had gone, had my examination, and left. My hospital visits were exercises in politeness. From time to time, I took the X rays and results of tests to my other doctor. No further need for the "small extra treatment" he had spoken of at the start. Everything was fine except for my material situation, which was as dependably precarious as it had always been. Highs, lows, very highs, very lows, one step forward, one step backward, two steps forward, two steps backward: stability of a sort. Some people are bored with life. I've never had the time or the means.

During this period, my career was trapped in an obstacle course I'd begun two years before which took me to the many ORTF offices scattered all over Paris. They were staffed by amiable people, and as interchangeable as cabinet members. They waltzed from one department to another at the whim of authorities all the more frightening for being imprecise, and whose overriding concern was never to take responsibility for anything. The race required a sound constitution, unremitting obstinacy, the faith of a zealot, and the influence of some well-placed friends. I made it, with what I can honestly describe as some success. But all too soon, I found myself back at the starting line with a new course to run and, just to screw me up, the hurdles in new places. One step forward, one step backward.

And why should I be in a greater hurry than the next man? Because I had cancer? No. Cancer gave me no claim to a higher priority, any more than it imbued me with greater talent, if I had any at all. It wouldn't do to have my literary agent, and friend, submit the comedy I had written after my operation and say to a prospective producer or theater director:

"It's a very funny piece; besides, the man who wrote it has cancer."

Funny and cancerous are unlikely bedfellows in the entertainment world, and a sick man is by definition sad and incapable of writing anything funny. It's a notion that's hard to combat. If my agent were to add, "The author is also very rich," which was not yet the case, the prospect might consider me an exception to the rule. He might then be expecting gallows humor, and would be disappointed to find that it was the work of a writer more concerned with making people laugh than with the anarchy in his cells.

My professional life was back where it had always been, and so was my private life. I seemed to offer my family extravagant dreams nourished by my work rather than the bourgeois comforts that bring harmony to the hearth. With the deepest affection, I offered them the castles in Spain I was always building, which regularly crumbled, burying me in rubble and a new load of debts. But I bounced right back with new projects certain of success which I wanted more for my family than for myself. It was a rare day that didn't bring me some measure of joy, and a measure of worry. But the latter comes readily. Everybody has that. Having said as much, I shouldn't be credited with a wisdom I don't possess and never will. Wisdom based on experience and reflection is not for me. It would produce only the calculated satisfactions suitable to reasonable people, and I am seldom reasonable.

I passed up the vow to stop drinking, thinking one sacrifice at a time enough and tobacco the more difficult. It wasn't long before I moved from soda water and tomato juice back to stronger stuff. Very soon, without even being aware of it, I was drinking as I had before: one day, several days, even weeks, nothing; then a little, a lot, too much, much too much. I don't do anything in moderation. A chance encounter, a special occasion, nerves, boredom with the eternal solitude that is the writer's lot. . . . There is no end to excuses for drinking.

In the fleeting euphoria of my television glory, I had said "fuck off" to the slave driver for whom I'd been producing endless comic strips designed for children but more often read by retarded adults. But when prospective buyers for my more elevated projects failed to bite, I began to wonder what had happened to the giddy rise I had expected after my first success. My faith in my future was no whit diminished, but it meant waiting. Then rescue came in the form of an old friend who hired me as a reader in his department at ORTF. Thanks to the minuscule and not very dependable salary he was able to pay, I found myself back on Social Security.

About the middle of the following January, the doctor who checked the results of my blood tests and X rays made a face as he took in the proportions of my unclothed body.

"Your tests are fine, but you are getting positively obese. We'll have to watch that."

I left with a diet in hand, the suggestion that I lay off the booze, and an appointment to come in six months later and several pounds lighter, for new tests and X rays.

Two weeks later, I woke up to find my neck surprisingly swollen. Had it been on the side the surgeon had trimmed off, it would have been an almost pleasant surprise: symmetry would have been reestablished. Unfortunately, this was not the case. The swelling was on the other side. It was large and virtually painless, but it looked very odd. I had my wife examine the phenomenon, and she made the prudent observation:

"You must have caught a chill in the night."

Coward that I am, I gladly accepted the good sense of her remark. I have the perhaps indecent habit of sleeping in the buff with the windows wide open, and in the cold weather we'd been having, this result was plausible. It's quite common, I know, but it had never happened to me before. That's what bothered me and bothered my wife. There is always an interlude of hesitation, that dead time before you find the courage to look the truth in the face. It didn't take us many days to decide that this swollen gland, which had resisted all the usual household remedies, was not an innocent swollen gland. We didn't mention the word "cancer," but it was clear that we both had it increasingly on our minds. We had kidded ourselves with, "It doesn't look like . . . there's no comparison with . . . the last tests were fine. . . ." You can't go on with that kind of pretending for very long unless you're an idiot. There was only one step to take, and one evening I took it.

Feeling that once again I'd better lose no time, I went to see my nose and throat man at his home.

"Doctor, you don't think my . . . that that damn thing is starting up again?" (Cancer is a forbidden word between doctor and patient.)

My haste was well understood. With a troubled look on his face, he gave me a protracted examination.

"After three years," he murmured, "this would really be tough luck. We'll try to get rid of the inflammation, but if we don't succeed, we'll have to do something else. But I'm sure we'll succeed.

"Thank you, Doctor." I smiled, but he didn't.

The next day, I was initiated into the delights of Propidon shots. Anyone who has experienced them knows how they can make the shortest month of the year seem like the longest. The swelling went down, went up, went down again. . . . The moment I woke up in the morning, I played the game of "are you there or aren't you?" It didn't interfere with my work, but it was taking up too much room among my preoccupations. It must have preoccupied the doctor too, for one morning I received a very nice letter from his colleague in hematology who had been informed of the "persistant glandular growth" and who invited me to come see him.

From that moment on, I had few illusions about the nature of my variable swelling. After a long period of playing possum, my cancer was back. A cancer is very wily: it plays dead, it thwarts the most astute medical treatment, then suddenly it reappears when you least expect it.

Two weeks later, after a series of tests and examinations, I received a second letter from the doctor, as bland as the first:

"I have just written Doctor X to ask him to excise a small gland in the region of your lower right maxillary. I think it is the wise thing to do. I would like to see you in a month. . . .

"Yours very sincerely. . . ."

I was learning how to read between the lines. My cancer had moved from one side of my neck to the other. Tacking from port to starboard, it had moved from one gland to another, keeping always to the same area of my lymphatic system. In a way, its affection for this particular region of my anatomy was encouraging. My cancer was no adventurer.

On my next visit to the hospital, the doctor who had operated on me before said in a soft voice that seemed a shade wearier than before:

"We'll operate whenever you like. It's for you to decide."

"Will the operation be as extensive as the first?"

The doctor made a vague gesture, leaving me free to draw my own conclusions: "I won't know until I operate." This was no cause for jubilation. I was going to be an archaeological site, with the doctor making a careful inventory of the digs.

"I don't need to see you again before the operation. When you've decided on the date, let the head nurse know and I'll operate the day after you're admitted."

I was beginning to know my doctor, so, realizing I'd get nothing more out of him, I got up to leave.

"Thank you, Doctor."

"And don't wait six months!" he said, with more worry than threat in his voice.

"You can count on me, Doctor."

We looked at each other. I'm sure he was aware that I understood far more than he had told me.

Once out of the hospital, I stopped for a drink at the first bistro that seemed suitable for meditation. After noon, there aren't too many empty bars in Paris, but I found one without the usual clientele taking a few moments off from work, and without that modern contraption that brays out the hits of the day. The absence of jukebox and clientele must have been related. The higher the decibel count, the happier people are; it starts in nursery school. Either this bartender was too old and not with it, or he had sensitive ears. Whichever it was, I was very grateful for the silence. I was there to make my peace with the inevitable.

It didn't take long. I had adopted a certain position relative to my cancer, and it couldn't be changed. Consistency played into my sense of dignity. Since I'd been brave once, without too much effort, I would be brave again. In any event, I was trapped, and relieved of the opportunity to hesitate. The thought of a second operation didn't bother me. Only, what kind of operation would it be? There the doctor had left me in the dark. In that phrase "excise a small gland," I caught a whiff of one of those lies doctors love to fall back on. I hadn't forgotten that tube in my nose. So, before going to the head nurse, I decided to see what more I could find out. If one doctor wouldn't be specific, the other might. The trick was to have an intermediary ask the question.

That very evening, my wife, somewhat reluctant but sensitive to my natural curiosity, telephoned the second doctor and spoke to him as I listened in.

"Doctor, is this just a simple excision of a gland, or will the operation be as serious as the last one?"

"Probably as serious, I would imagine."

"You really think so?"

"Yes, but I don't think I'd tell your husband."

I smiled. I had found out what I wanted to know.

I knew what to expect, approximately. Equally approximately, I made my own diagnosis of my case using all the encyclopedias and dictionaries in the house, buttressed by my own vivid imagination. It was obvious that my lymphatic system was the locus of my cancer, but it was a long step between a lymphosarcoma and Hodgkin's disease, a step my limited knowledge forbade me to take. Something was going on in my lymphatic system which had for the time being become localized in the cervical region, and that's all I needed to know. Had I been able to give my cancer a more precise definition, it would have become like all the others in that category, depersonalized, anybody's cancer, and I wouldn't stand for that. My cancer was unique of its kind, a made-to-order cancer, to fit me, be like me. Meaning a nice cancer.

My admission to the hospital was scheduled for Palm Sunday. One less pilgrim on the road to Rome. I put my affairs, such as they were, in order and told the few people who might be interested that I'd be out of circulation for two weeks which, at that time of year, sounded like a school vacation.

Granted I could have done without this new trip to the hospital, I was determined not to dramatize. There were plenty of people to do that for me: "cancer . . . relapse . . . metastasis . . . operation . . . treatments. . . ." Many saw it as an inauspicious omen, some as the end. I used my last few days to reinforce my morale, even—I say it without shame—to provoking my friends' appreciation of my undaunted courage.

"You really are admirable!" "If I were in your shoes, I

don't know if I could. . . ." "There aren't many people like you!"

With such comments as these, a poor slob feels transported to higher levels, and capable of outdoing even himself. To use the current phrase, I was psyching myself up.

Saturday night, my wife and older son—the younger one was shivering somewhere in England—and I had dinner in a Chinese restaurant in the Latin Quarter after going to Fellini's *The Clowns*. I love clowns, and I love that *quartier* of vivid memories. I also love *langoustines en beignets* and all those dishes that not only delight the palate but give the added joy of taking you to distant places. The evening worked out well.

The next day, at the hour when parishioners, their Sunday duty done, file out of church, I went in. Once again, piling up all the odds in my favor, I asked the small solitary flame to bring me light and protect me. I picked up a few palm fronds, left my donation in the box, and rushed to the neighborhood betting booth. Like most middle-class Frenchmen, I'm more generous with the nags than with our poor struggling priests. Matins may gain you paradise, but that comes much later. And it hasn't been proved for sure.

Even though the day's races were not the only reason for my visit to church, I couldn't help inserting a timid request to the Lord that he bring my three horses home the way I picked them. It would be a big help. Perhaps my request failed for want of discretion, for it was only partially granted; two out of the three horses came in, like most other people's. God is just. At five that afternoon, my wife accompanied me to the hospital. It was a dull, gray day. It usually is on Palm Sunday.

My bed was in a room like the one I'd had before, but

this time I didn't have to fear a trunk. I had found out my program of novelties didn't include one this time.

As soon as I arrived, I was struck by the strange appearance of the roommate I had drawn. He was a small man, wallowing in a pair of pajamas much too large for him, and his face was curiously heavy around the jaws, reminding me of someone, but who? "Have you noticed Popeye?" my wife asked under her breath as she was helping me get installed. That's who it was! Popeye! All he was missing was the pipe and Popeye's gaiety, for this one was clearly not having a good time.

Once my wife had put everything in order, there was nothing left for her but to go. We had said all there was to say; anything more would have been useless, even embarrassing. Fortunately, she felt the same way.

We separated at the top of a dimly lit staircase, like school stairs on a Sunday night. (I'd spent many years in boarding school and knew that such petty economies were one of the justifications of school administrations.) I heard the door close two flights below and went back to my room.

The man I was to share it with, having priority over me, had already made himself at home.

"There've been two men here before you, two were operated on like me, two have left, but I'm still here. They seem to want to keep me here. If you leave before they let me out. . . ."

Then he poured out everything that was weighing on his soul. Why were they keeping him longer than the others? It was profoundly unjust. He seemed to take his protracted stay as some sort of hoax, for which he blamed the doctors, not his illness. He had only one idea in his head, to get out of the hospital. He had gone from hospital to hospital, from treatment to cure, from cure to operation, and he was sick of the whole thing. He was down to eighty-six pounds; these he wanted to keep at all costs, and the only way was to get out of this room, go home, go to a convalescent home, go anywhere but here. It wasn't for me to explain that diseases were unfair. Besides, did he have any idea what his disease was? Hadn't he guessed, with everything he had gone through and all those he'd seen at close range, that what he had was cancer? I don't think so. There are different states of grace.

After a dinner I barely touched, and he even less, I tried to read, but I couldn't concentrate. A few visitors stopped by, then the ward was prepared for the night. I went and watched a dull movie on television. Not being sleepy, I was the last to leave. As I wandered back to my room, I was surprised to see a strange-looking vehicle pulled up near the landing. With its cotton hood, it looked like a very long baby buggy. I peered inside. It was made of zinc, like an outsized rain gutter. What for? In a nearby room, behind a screen which hid little, men in white were quietly busying themselves around a body. Now I understood: the superbuggy was for him.

"I arrive, another leaves," I said to myself as I lay in bed. I've never been affected by death, and the sleeping pills I'd been given were taking effect. I had a good night's sleep.

The next morning my old friend stopped by with his wagon.

"Are you here again?"

"That's right."

He wrapped me in a blanket with all the care of a young mother, and off we went. As we were rolling along, he announced solemnly:

"I don't like Mondays. Monday isn't a good day. I'm not in good shape on Mondays."

I said: "Do you think I like Monday?"

He laughed; he hadn't thought of that.

"Well, your morale seems good, anyway."

My morale was good enough, but once I was strapped to the operating table, I wanted things to get going. Where was everybody? There were no nurses around; perhaps they were operating in another room. Yes, I could see that Monday wasn't a good day.

As the minutes dragged on, my much-touted morale began to crumble. All kinds of thoughts entered my head: if the attendant wasn't in good shape on Mondays, maybe the anesthetist wasn't, or the surgeon; maybe both? A tiring visit to the country, a long dinner, a late return home; there are lots of reasons for feeling tired on Monday. It doesn't take much to make the eye a little less sharp, the hand less steady. A distraction, a sudden motion—my preoperation movie was starting up again. Then a very small thing brought me back to reality: I needed to scratch my nose.

I tried to dismiss the need while it was still vague and bearable, for with my hands strapped down I couldn't do anything about it. I told myself that my nose wasn't really bothering me, that I didn't really need to scratch it, that it would go away by itself. But instead, the need grew stronger and stronger: first it was irritating, then it became an obsession, then torture. It took hold of me from head to foot. I was one raging desire to scratch my nose. It was ludicrous and agonizing at the same time. Finally I had to plead for mercy:

"Nurse, nurse . . ."

Since I couldn't see anything but the operating room light above me, I was calling into the unknown.

"What's the matter?" a woman's voice said close to me.

"Nurse, will you for God's sake scratch my nose?"

There are moments when a man isn't very proud of himself. Yet the invisible nurse found my uncontrollable panic perfectly natural.

"Gladly," she said in a noncommittal tone, and went to work. Well scratched and delivered of my agony, I could only feel shame. I tried to find an excuse for my silly behavior.

"It's pretty stupid, isn't it?" I said, trying to smile.

"Why stupid?"

The conversation stopped there. I remember nothing more. Nothing until I was rudely awakened by a volley of slaps—the house specialty. The energetic woman was good at her job, but I did wonder why, since the technique of putting a patient to sleep had made such progress, the method of waking him up was still so primitive.

I took in the fact that I was in bed and that I didn't have a tube in my nose. If I said more, it would be pure invention. Memory, or at least mine, doesn't register everything equally: it takes in certain things in sharp detail and skips others, often the most important. It's my luck to have a selective memory that carefully preserves what I want to remember, even the most useless details of my distant past, and rejects what is best forgotten. My memory rejects a great deal. It is a benign memory.

The next day, everything went as it should. I was up for a little while; I did the crossword puzzle; I had some visitors, as did Popeye; I read a few pages of the book I'd begun before the operation; and that evening, I drew a surprised and somewhat irritated reaction from the orderly who had come to take my blood pressure.

"Two hundred and sixty." he exclaimed, looking at me as if I were trying to put something over on him. He repeated the operation twice. It was plain that I was being perverse and that it must be made to come down.

· The next morning, I had another unpleasant surprise. As I was brushing my teeth, I suddenly noticed that my tongue was acting strangely. It was on the bias.

"What the hell did they do this time?" I fumed. "Why doesn't it work the way it used to?"

I directed it right, left, up, down. There was no getting around it: my tongue was askew. What had they done to me? With great speed and logic, I asked myself the next question:

"Is my tongue crooked just for now, or forever?"

These two alternatives, particularly the one affecting my future, amply filled the morning. Sitting in a chair between Popeye's bed and mine, a book in my hand to give me a look of composure, I tested the agility of my tongue with my mouth closed as the blackest thoughts raced through my head. From time to time, I got up and looked at it in the mirror. No discernible change. When the medical student who was making the doctor's rounds that morning stopped by, I let him have it. Had he been the doctor, I would have been more guarded, but with a mere student, I expressed myself freely. What had they done to my tongue? The student could hardly be held responsible for the results of an operation he had witnessed only from a distance, but he seemed flattered that I should ask. He launched into a long and meticulous explanation: they had been forced to dig much deeper than anticipated and had cut into a jugular vein, a very delicate and complicated operation. My instructor ticked off an unending series of things he had seen, things he said would have made my flesh creep, things I wouldn't have been able to stand, things I was so lucky I hadn't seen. . . .

"They touched a nerve, but they didn't damage it. It isn't damaged at all," he said with great conviction.

[56]

Not damaged! Perhaps I should have thanked him, maybe congratulated him? My tongue was paralyzed on one side, but the nerve had not been damaged! What more could you ask for without seeming ungrateful?

"You think it will take care of itself?" I ventured.

"Of course, since the nerve wasn't . . ."

Then he was off again. My anger gradually subsided and gave way to weariness and a touch of sympathy. This future doctor, hiding his youth under a well-trimmed beard, was being very kind and showing great interest in my case. He was already talking with the assurance of an experienced doctor, well practiced in the art of lying. Clearly, he had a talent for his chosen profession.

He promised that a specialist would stop by to look into my blood pressure problem and left me, protesting that everything was going exactly as it should. Then he turned to Popeye and told him exactly what he'd told me. This was too much. Maybe I was wrong; appearances can lie. But looking at Popeye, I wouldn't have bet much on his recovery.

The first week went by very quickly. Books, treatments, visits, meals, books. . . . In a hospital, you get into a certain rhythm and let yourself go; the days carry you along without your making any effort. On Easter Sunday there was a great pealing of bells. On Tuesday my stitches were removed, and I was able to take in the proportions of my new neck. Very curious indeed. My head was still the same old head, but the neck holding it up didn't seem to be mine. I took it in slowly, trying not to remember. From acceptance, I moved to criticism: my new neck was a poor thing, and symmetry was the least of its virtues. On the other hand, the "jugular" side was not, relatively speaking, as bad as the other. Then, as I had with my tongue, I put my neck through a series of exercises. I could turn it reasonably well; it could move forward, backward, almost as well as its predecessor, and if it pulled a bit, it must be that it needed breaking in. And, like a pair of new shoes, it pinched a little. All it needed was use. I would get used to it. In a manner of speaking, we would each get used to the other.

I was to leave the hospital on Friday. Thursday morning I went downstairs for my last consultation. My wife had asked to be there, and even though I would have preferred otherwise, I didn't oppose her. After all, the worst was behind me. At least, that's what I thought when I sat down opposite the doctor. Next to him stood his colleague who was going to be in charge of my radiotherapy treatments at another hospital.

The first doctor described in detail the work he had performed on my modest person. Most of it was beyond my comprehension, but I did gather that he was satisfied. Therefore I must be too, and out of politeness, I acted like a blissful fool who is proud of having been an ideal patient.

"Please open your mouth," he said, after having examined its exterior.

I obeyed, and that is when things took a bad turn.

"But he has his teeth!" the second doctor exclaimed.

What was so strange about that? Of course I had teeth, not all of them obviously, and not too many in good shape, but I was grateful for those I had, including the stumps. They were like old servants, not very handsome but useful all the same.

"They have to come out. All of them. It's essential."

Pull out all my teeth? Whatever for?

"You really think so?" the first doctor asked.

"Absolutely. I have to get way up there, in order to get in here, and here. Otherwise we risk necrosis."

Pointing out the parts of my face and neck to be x-rayed, he went after my teeth. He had no trouble bringing the other doctor around, and even today I wonder if they weren't in collusion. Doctors have more than one trick in their black bags.

"So?" The surgeon looked at me with a certain compassion.

I felt crestfallen, and must have looked it.

"If we must, we must," I said, with little enthusiasm.

"Perhaps you'd prefer to go home for a few days, then come back."

"No. Since it has to be done and I'm here, let's get it over with as soon as possible."

The decision was made quickly. The extraction would take place under general anesthetic the following morning, and I could go home on Saturday. The radiotherapy would begin the week after. That seemed to me far off and of little importance.

"Well, that's it, then," the surgeon said. "I guess I'm through with you. There is nothing more I can take out. Good day."

We shook hands and I thanked him. I also shook hands with the doctor who was going to take out my teeth and who was giving me a big toothy smile, the bastard. As we reached the deserted waiting room, we exchanged a few joyless words, and the doctor said as he left:

"I'd give up the whiskey if I were you." (That's the kind of advice women like.) "See you Tuesday."

I don't think we answered him. My wife was too busy feeling sorry for me, and I couldn't find anything to say. I told her to go home for lunch. Not much consolation, but a reasonable suggestion. It was late. She left and I went back up to my room. I found Popeye, if not joyful—he was no longer capable of that—at least less morose. He was leaving the next day. I congratulated him. I was happy for him. As happy as you can be when your head is full of teeth.

For that's all I had in my head. Teeth! My teeth! My teeth and me, and me without my teeth. First without teeth, then with a denture. Some ideas are harder to accept than others. The idea of wearing a denture came very hard.

A denture; false teeth. False teeth are for farces and gags. The fount of funny stories and hilarious comic strips, the unquenchable source of jokes and belly laughs. Always your neighbor's, of course. Never for a second had I ever imagined that such a humiliating calamity could befall me. I'm still a child much of the time, which must have been the reason for the instinctive repulsion, the childish fear for my sad dental future. Sad? Well, I don't like having my future imposed on me.

I soon directed my thoughts back to something more suitable to my present age. Thinking it over, my dental future wasn't all that bad. For one thing, I'd be completely unconscious during the extractions and wouldn't feel a thing. Anyone who has ever had a tooth pulled needs only to multiply it by the total number of teeth in his head to understand the agony I was escaping. Another comfort was the progress in the dental arts. The era of false teeth worn only for great occasions was well behind us. We were now in the age of "implants" and invisible "prostheses."

How things change when you make the simple effort of changing their names! False teeth, even a denture— no! A prosthesis? Why not? Beautiful people, people in the news, many of them wear prostheses and no one is any the wiser. I ticked off the well-publicized smiles of the top luminaries in the world of arts and letters and wondered how many of them owed their dazzling teeth to the work of a talented prosthetist. Then, coming down a peg, I considered some of my friends. I arrived at some very consoling conclusions.

A lady anesthetist came to see me during the course of the afternoon.

"Well, I'm told I'm to put you to sleep tomorrow," she said, and examined the information sheet attached to the foot of my bed.

"So I'm told," I said, with some reserve, remembering the cuffing I'd be getting to wake me up. As she was reading the list of drugs I was given daily, she suddenly exclaimed:

"But I can't do it! They're giving you"—I've forgotten the name—"for your blood pressure. If I put you to sleep, you'll never wake up again."

"I don't like that at all!" I said vehemently. "I have no intention of dying!"

"Don't worry," she said with an encouraging smile. "We'll give you a local anesthesia."

Local anesthesia! Good God! I knew what that meant. I started counting my teeth. For the first, and last, time I regretted that I still had so many. Even giving it the benefit of the doubt, tomorrow's session promised to be long.

But what if the anesthetist hadn't come to see me? What would have happened? The conviction returned that I was lucky, something I had mistakenly begun to doubt. Given what I had—my cancer—what did a handful of teeth matter? Nor were my teeth new; they were old, they had given me long service, but they would inevitably give me trouble some time in the future. All in all, it wasn't such a bad idea to be rid of the lot. Back in the days when I had my milk teeth, it would have been cause for rejoicing. Before going to sleep, I would have slipped them under my pillow, and the little mouse, or fairy—depending on your beliefs—would have taken them away while I was asleep and left me, in view of the number, a very large present. Too bad: the little mouse, or fairy, had long since lost interest in me. Why do these pleasant rites atrophy with age? A tooth is a tooth, dammit!

His back to me, Popeye was emptying his drawers and celebrating his imminent departure with great tact. I picked up my book and tried to read.

If Mondays were not good days, Fridays were apparently little better. When my wagon-pushing friend came for me, he was in a great hurry.

"We've got a real heavy day today," he said. "I'll take you down now, but you may have to wait around a while."

He addressed me as if I were a man who would understand. I felt flattered. He was treating me like an old customer, not as someone just in off the street. Stretched out on the wagon, I felt a little sleepy from the shot I'd been given. I waited patiently in the hall for an operating room to be free. I was pretty unconscious, but I do remember a lot of people milling around, wagons rolling this way and that. Then my turn came.

I'm sorry in a way that I recall so little of what followed. If I hadn't been so fuzzy in the head, I could have learned a great deal. From the voices around me, I gathered that the stomatologist in charge was teaching a group of students. A woman's hand, anonymous as before, held mine, and the demonstration of which I was the subject began: "I'm going to stick the needle in here, which corresponds to . . ."

It didn't always correspond on the first attempt; this much I knew. Comatose as I was, I could hear the doctor's explanations, feel the needles, hear metallic noises, extractions, more shots, more explanations. "My, my, they're still using pink thread!" Why pink thread? I was paying less and less attention when suddenly the operating room light was turned out, and the operation was over. I had joined the kingdom of the armadillo, anteater, and sloth, the elite of the toothless. I was no longer an elephant; I had made new associations in the animal world.

The end of that day is a complete fog. I was dimly aware of Popeye's departure, which I acknowledged with the grunt of a wounded beast.

The next day, lucid once again, I made an inventory. Seen from the outside, I had the battered face of a boxer, winner or loser, it mattered little, who had left his mouthpiece in the locker room. When I opened my mouth, fear gave way to astonishment. It wasn't as awful as I expected, but it was certainly strange. The "pink thread" had been used to sew up my gums. What prodigies of science! I looked like a rolled roast in a butcher's window. Something told me it was time I left this hospital.

Early that afternoon, and in unbecoming haste, I took my 176 pounds home. As with Popeye before me, I was convinced that distance was my refuge. Refuge from what? The reason a dog retreats to the doghouse is to lick his wounds.

3

Once I was back in my familiar nest, there was nothing
to do but wait. I knew it would be two months before
my dentist could install temporary choppers. Sixty
toothless days may not spell a man's doom, but it did
suggest certain inconveniences and the end of gas-
tronomy as I had known it. Still and all, I was fat enough
to tolerate some abstinence. A man can live on two
quarts of milk a day, not with delight, perhaps, but he
can live. The return to infancy suited me well enough,
especially since I didn't slobber and could talk. By keeping my mouth almost completely shut and taking my
time, I could express myself quite normally—to those
who didn't know me. So long as I didn't get angry or
laugh, no one could guess that my tongue was askew and
my gums ungarnished. There is no beauty without some
suffering. And so, for the sake of appearances, and to
preserve my tender self-esteem, I forced myself to keep a
tight rein on my voluble temperament.

A new ascot around my neck, I set out Sunday morning for a stroll around my neighborhood. My absence

had probably gone unnoticed. I have no public or daily function like the postman, milkman, or garbage collector. When these men don't show up, people notice it: it affects their lives; they comment on it. I was only part of the scenery; people greeted me, talked to me, but forgot me the moment I disappeared, for I served no essential function. What use is a writer? Be that as it may, over the years I had made a number of friends in my neighborhood, which made it a sort of a village, with all the good things that implies.

It wasn't a very long walk. Just time enough to buy a newspaper, shake a few hands, exchange a word here and there, pay my Sunday homage to the pari-mutuel booth, and return home a little more confident, a little stronger. Stronger for having heard certain words, seen the surprised expression on a few faces in which I read a hint of admiration, probably more than was really there, but no matter. I was playing a little game. I hadn't gone out because I "wanted a breath of fresh air," as I told my wife with studied casualness—she having less reason to believe me than most—but to garner a little sympathy as yet another reward for good behavior.

Courage, like beauty, is a courtesan: to blossom, it needs to be noticed, to be complimented. Courage needs support. Unfortunately, the military have long known this, and the man who invented medals was no fool, much as I deplore his initiative. "Private Smith, I hereby decorate you for bravery." Smith is a happy fellow; he is proud, people are looking at him, they applaud, he sticks out his chest. Smith is a hero. Poor bastard, he's been trapped, and his stupid medal is a life sentence without appeal. The next time he's sent off to war, even though he may loathe the prospect, Private Smith must live up to his reputation. Scared or not, he must march forward.

His attitude to danger has been decided for him. Should he suddenly stop being brave, no one would understand; he would be accused of cowardice. Everybody knows that a hero never falters.

I'm no hero. And in the battle against disease, the doctors get the decorations, not the patients. So I have to set my own booby trap; I wouldn't want anybody to see me falter.

Early the next Tuesday, we appeared at the hospital where I was to have the radiotherapy treatments. I say we because my wife insisted on coming and I didn't have the heart to stop her. We followed the signs until we reached the room where I was to find my doctor. We waited, my wife far more apprehensive than I. I had interrogated Popeye on the subject; he had had a big dose, but he said it hadn't bothered him. "You don't feel a thing," he'd said. This would have been more reassuring had it not come from such a scrawny patient. Where had Popeye lost all that weight? Here, probably. Maybe not all of it, but a large part. I wasn't against losing weight so long as it was kept within reason. Finally my turn came.

The doctor greeted us with his broad smile, which I no longer held against him. After a few general comments, he summoned the technician who was to take me in charge. Using a large red crayon, the doctor marked out the area on my skin that she was to radiate, together with some technical observations I didn't understand. I have no talent for the so-called exact sciences, and I didn't like the idea of being part of an algebraic equation in which I would be playing the role of the unknown factor. Naked from the waist up, chest out, lips closed, and belly flattened (as much as I could), I let myself be daubed with the stoicism of a well-brought-up child. To be naked in front of people wearing clothes is an art in itself: you're always afraid you haven't washed thoroughly; maybe an odor . . .?

"There!" The artwork was done, and the doctor smiled at his handiwork. Then he added, not for my benefit, "Don't forget to protect his larynx."

Now the doctor was back on my level. These were words I could understand, and I was grateful. The fact that my larynx was going to be protected was good news. The word brought to mind its function. It was my voice they were going to protect, and my voice is more than just another part of my anatomy. For better or worse, my voice is a very important part of me, of my personality.

The administrative formalities were dispatched with alacrity—given a little luck and consideration, this is actually possible. I waited my turn for the treatment. There were a number of us, but as far as I was concerned, all we had in common was the waiting. I rejected with all my soul the idea that we belonged to the same family. Many of them were obviously very ill, had even come here in ambulances. An ambulance is a piece of medical equipment that fools nobody: after that vehicle comes the hearse. Circumstances would soon be ridding me of that simplistic assumption, but that morning I was still blessed with the stubborn optimism that disaster might strike others but never me. It was a positive relief to hear my name called.

As I undressed once again, I cast an unfriendly eye on the panel in the control room. That's where it was all determined: the quantity of rays that would slyly infiltrate my body. I was ready to admit that one insidious evil could be used to fight another, but that my fate should be decided, even for a second, by needles trotting around a predetermined course, left me with a disagreeable sensation. Man's nature is often at war with progress.

With my shirt off, I was able to admire the doctor's art in the mirror of my cubicle. The color of the crayon and the primitive scrawl made me look like an Indian. I had symmetrical zebra stripes from my cheeks to my chin, and my scars were handsomely framed to bring out their best. I was wondering if they would be hard to remove when I heard my name called again.

While the technician changed the white paper on the table, I took a long hard look at the mysterious contraption hovering over the table. I felt the same distrust as a chicken going into the oven. Rays cooked you too, they could even burn you and burn horribly; well-intentioned people had told me so.

"Please lie down on your left side."

The young women placed me in a comfortable position, my nose buried in a pillow, pushed the table, made various adjustments, turned my head a little more, made more adjustments, pulled my shoulder back, checked the whole, and finally, to my great relief, placed a big piece of lead across my larynx, held in place by a glass support.

"Now, don't move until I tell you."

The door closed. Seconds passed. There was complete silence. Then a motor suddenly started humming above me. I held my breath while my heart knocked against my ribs. Popeye hadn't lied; I didn't feel a thing. Yet something had happened. Something was going on inside me that I wasn't aware of. My one available eye took in a pretty postcard tacked on the otherwise bare wall while my mind snatched at visions of atom bombs falling on Japan. The idea of getting overcooked began to haunt me. I could do one of two things: pray or count. The extent of the danger did not seem to justify prayer, so I started counting. I counted like a man possessed. I had passed four hundred when the motor stopped abruptly. It was over. I had come through the first session unharmed.

Once up, I walked over to the postcard I'd been eyeing so long.

"What a pretty place!" I said gamely.

I didn't give a damn about the place, but I wanted to show that I appreciated the attempt to humanize this scene of misery. What thoughtful person had had the idea? Someone who had been here? Someone who had lain on that table? No matter. True charity is anonymous, and the best kind is collective.

"Very pretty," I said again, and turned toward the young woman who was already readying the table for the next patient.

"Yes, isn't it," she said politely.

"Do the people who come here usually know what's wrong with them?"

I had kept asking myself that question in the waiting room, and she was the only person around who could give me an answer. She was not expecting it, and for a fraction of a second, she stopped adjusting the paper toweling and looked at me:

"No," she said, and resumed her work. She obviously didn't like the question, and besides, she was in a hurry. From my cubicle, I heard her call out another name. She was a fast worker. Minutes were precious: there were so many still waiting.

Before I left, the technician weighed me and wrote a figure down on a grim gray card on which she had written my name, the date, and the hour of treatment. I was to bring it back at each session. The number of lines, front and back, was intimidating. The days and days I would be returning. . . .

"Don't wash your neck," she said. "Just take a sponge bath. You must be very careful not to irritate your skin with soap and water."

"What about the red crayon on my cheeks?"

"Oh, you mustn't touch those! We'll do a delineation of the field tomorrow. Good-bye."

Delineation of the field? What in God's name could that be? I adjusted my ascot—the red in it went very well with the color of the crayon on my cheeks—and left to find my wife.

"How did it go?" she asked.

"Very well."

For once, I wasn't lying. Others were being driven away in ambulances; I was on my own two feet. All the same, a little farther along, we hailed a taxi.

"Treatments for patients who fail to appear at the appointed hour will be permanently cancelled." The warning was clear and unambiguous, and when I read it at the bottom of the card the technician had handed me, it came as a shock. It was clearly aimed at me. Clocks and I have never gotten along, and that word "permanently" filled me with foreboding. "Appointed hour" and "cancelled" were printed in bold type to underscore the sin and its punishment. Those three words carried the impact of a threat, and I knew its reach: if you're not on time, no more treatments, no more hope of a cure. Despite its Prussian tone, I understood the need for the warning. There were always more and more people waiting in line.

But what if I hadn't been warned? What if, like the others, I didn't know I had cancer? Knowing myself as I do, I didn't wish to dwell on those possibilities. So, the next morning, I arrived at the "appointed hour," unbathed and probably a bit smelly, the red crayon marks a little less vivid from having rubbed off on my pillow during the night. Actually, I was over twenty minutes early. What fear will do to a man!

I went through the formalities at the cashier's window, the newspaper, the crossword puzzle; and finally my name was called out. I must go here for X rays, there for a blood sample, to still another place for the "delineation of the field"; only then would I be ready for radiotherapy. My head full of topographical directions, I set off on my journey and its designated stops, a kind of hopscotch in a hospital setting. A little blood left here, X rays taken there, I reached the last square—my "delineation."

This was the domain of two women, one the doctor, the other a student. Once again I undressed to the waist, and graciously submitted to the request that I turn this way and that, face this machine and that one, while trying to figure out what it was all about. The ladies' concentration made conversation difficult. It would have been unseemly to distract them with such a childish question as "What are you doing that for?" Besides, they probably wouldn't have answered me. Isn't it a waste of time to explain what you're doing if the patient doesn't know what ails him?

"Now lie down there, please."

"There" was a wooden table with, at one end, a semicircle sprouting long spikes like knitting needles— something between a guillotine and a sideshow booth. Once my neck was strapped in place, I realized that instead of being there to pierce my neck, their function was to measure it. The doctor could have had the grace to tell me. . . .

"Don't move," she said as she approached me with a syringe containing a dark liquid. "I'm going to prick you."

With that thing! What was she doing to me? Once on the right side. Turn your head. Once on the left. Done.

"You may get up now. I'll see you tomorrow."

Indifferent to my tastes in the matter, she had tattooed me like a sailor. My neck was embellished with two blue, and indelible, almost symmetrical marks. So that was a "delineation of the field"! I returned to the radiotherapy room, had my daily dose, and went home with the awful knowledge that I would be back at that hospital, at the same hour, the next day, and the day after, for weeks and weeks. No one had told me how long the treatments were to go on.

Saturdays, Sundays, and holidays excepted, the monotony of my nonexistence was a computerized certainty. I say nonexistence because I retain only sporadic and disconnected memories of a period that bore precious little relation to life as lived to the fullest. Minutes, hours, even days escape my memory, hence my past. I always carry a diary which I use regularly: for this period, there isn't a name, an appointment, a telephone number. Nothing. Only white pages testifying to my absence from life.

Physically, I was present, but present only in relation to problems of nourishment, to my wayward saliva, and to the pesky concerns linked to my treatments. My brain, immobilized by these unaccustomed chores, had lost all its freedom. I simply wasn't there. All I retained of my old self was my unshakable belief in a better future. I was going through a bad time, but I knew for certain that I would get through it somehow. How was of no importance.

[72]

My old self peeked through a little when I left my apartment for the trip to the hospital. I put on my personality the way you put on a coat. I wanted to appear to others the way I myself felt. I was determined that nobody mistake the state of my health and class me too quickly among those referred to in the past tense. To anyone who asked, I said I was feeling fine, that no, radiotherapy was not tiring, that it was all a matter of patience. People smiled, looked pleased, and gave me words of encouragement that rang false. I wonder how many I convinced. Very few, I'm sure. It is hard to convince people that having cancer doesn't necessarily mean imminent death, especially when you're spending half your life shuttling back and forth to the hospital. "I thought you were a goner," one of them told me later. Pessimism comes easily when someone else is involved.

The pessimism I seemed to promote in others was given an unwelcome boost a few days later when, as I was leaving the hospital after my treatment, an ambulance driver called to me:

"I'm to take you home, sir."

"Why? I can go home perfectly well by myself."

"It's all arranged. No use tiring yourself for nothing."

"But I'm not that sick."

"Get in, get in. . . . This way."

Bewildered and humbled, I protested feebly as I let myself be shown into the ambulance waiting in the courtyard. Sitting comfortably next to the white-coated driver, I felt a tinge of superiority, which took on added dimensions when a guard raised the barrier at the entrance. I was one of the regulars.

Later on, when we found ourselves in heavy traffic, I was a little annoyed that the driver didn't use his siren. Not that I was in a hurry, but since I was in an ambulance, I wanted what was coming to me. I was exasperated with other drivers' lack of respect. Why doesn't that fool get out of the way? Doesn't he see us? The callousness of drivers is not to be believed! Had they lost all trace of humanity? My driver was of the same mind. He too was dismayed, but unfortunately he had no right to use his siren except when his charge was at death's door, and he was allowed to go full-blast with an escort of two motorcycles to clear the way.

He stepped on the gas, passed, braked, stepped on the gas again, all the while chatting with me and answering his radio calls. The man had the virtuosity of a racing car driver. When he deposited me outside my house, he said:

"We'll pick you up at quarter to ten tomorrow morning. Okay? Good-bye, sir."

I shook his hand, thanked him, and stepped down.

People were watching. I could easily guess what was going through their minds, with an ambulance picking me up and returning me every day at the same time. To make matters worse, I had felt obliged to tell everybody within shouting distance the nature of my illness. Not one person in a hundred would reasonably grant me more than the shortest reprieve.

But I soon learned to appreciate the great convenience of my ambulance, the greatest being that it relieved me of the necessity of keeping track of time. Even with that grim gray card, henceforth if I were late getting to the hospital, it would be the ambulance's fault.

That much said, I tried not to abuse my perquisites. I was ready when the ambulance arrived. In a matter of days I knew virtually every driver in the ambulance service. They were all cheerful and considerate young men, and I enjoyed talking to them when they had the time. Rushing to the bedside is supposedly one of golden rules of medicine, and the ambulance drivers never forgot this. In the middle of the worst traffic, the distant voice was there to remind them that every second counted, that Mr. A was to be picked up, then Mrs. B, and Miss C taken home. Flooring the accelerator was a duty, and if the passenger's stomach sometimes heaved, the driver's heart was in the right place.

Everything comes to an end, and one morning, I came to the last of my treatments. I had received my allotment of radium, and all that remained was to pick up the pieces after a six-weeks lapse. I was not in good shape. I had shed pounds, superfluous pounds to be sure, but my body missed them. My rear end drooped; the skin over my belly sagged; and my calves, once a source of pride during my holidays by the sea, had melted away. Instead of having firm and well-proportioned legs, I was reduced to matchsticks. Hideous!

To complement this ugliness, all signs of beard had disappeared from the radiated zone. Like Attila, where radium had been, nothing ever grew again. My "bayonet trench," once so difficult to shave, was gone for good. Fortunately, I have never equated hair with virility, so I was able to rejoice in the fact that the time spent with my razor was reduced by half. There's hardly a man alive who can't grasp that advantage.

When I went to see the surgeon the following Thursday, he must have found me a poor specimen. He immediately agreed with my radiologist that I should have a spell in the country before I embarked on the next stage of treatment as prescribed by the hematologist, that being chemotherapy. Leaving Paris just then was very inconvenient for me, but I knew the young doctor was bent on having me start the new treatment as soon as possible, and had even regretted not starting it right after my first operation. As a dutiful and trusting patient, I wished to oblige. My doctors were interested in my welfare, even when their recommendations did not always coincide. They finally hit on a compromise that suited me well. I would go to a convalescent home for a month and then start the new treatments as soon as I returned.

My fate thus determined, a social worker in the hospital set about finding the best place to answer my needs. It was not easy, for time was of the essence, and I was a very fussy bird when it came to the kind of cage I would let myself be cooped up in. She knew me well, having seen my wife more often than me, and took note of my conditions: that I have a room to myself, and that I be able to eat my meals in my room. I knew I had to eat. Now, eating in private was difficult enough; in public, it would have been indecent. I refused to make a spectacle of myself with my new denture, and I was not going to leave Paris without teeth. When I travel, I want to go whole.

It was not my usual dentist who took me in charge but a young assistant who explained that his boss had been hospitalized for several weeks with a serious liver condition. It was cancer, and he didn't know it. Was it better this way? Not to know? I wondered. I was not prepared to give a verdict where others were concerned. How could I know how I would react if I had their cancer instead of my own?

In any event, within eight days, my new set of teeth was ready. I took it for an airing before my departure and visited various offices where friends had been wondering about my long absence. I was glad to see them, we exchanged pleasantries, I was my usual self, even more so. They may well have thought that my gaiety didn't go with the way I looked, that perhaps I was overdoing it, but they had the tact not to say so.

What did bother me was the spray of saliva that suddenly glistened in the sunlight. By God, I was a walking sprinkler system! My twisted tongue and new teeth were getting along well enough separately, but their union required the strictest surveillance. In intimate conversation, I was a dangerous adversary. My thoughts tended to outrun my speech, and the result was often a hazardous splutter. Certain sounds were deformed, and a number of words had to be abandoned entirely. Unfortunately, they were the more colorful ones that I had long depended on to season my conversation. With expressiveness gone, civility increased, which is probably a good thing, though a little boring. I also had the impression that people were making fun of me. It isn't easy to shrug your shoulders and pass silently by, especially for me.

Unrepentant blabbermouth that I am, with these few exceptions, life went on as usual. Aesthetically speaking, my new teeth became me. That at least was my wife's "impartial" observation. "They aren't noticeable at all! No one would ever guess they weren't yours. . . ." I was more than ready to believe her, and set off for the mountain region selected for me with high anticipation. The country was new to me, and my mode of travel beyond my wildest expectations. So that I wouldn't have to undergo a long and tiring train trip, the hospital had provided an ambulance. I was heading toward restored health, the unknown, and in a private conveyance! Four hundred miles between me and my past, present, and future worries! I knew I was lucky, but not to that degree. . . .

The moment the ambulance left Paris and was speeding down the highway, I had an almost physical sensation of renewal. My brain, numb for weeks, began slowly turning over. I was living at seventy miles an hour, and I don't mean the speed of the ambulance but the ravenous appetite with which I wolfed down everything we passed. I was drunk on life, as if to make up for the time I had almost given it up. Life asks to be loved. Life deserves it; but you have to work to deserve it. When we ran into a sudden shower and the driver slowed down, I kept my eyes glued to the road. There was too much at stake to tolerate even the thought of an accident.

My joy in the trip was further enhanced by the driver, who knew the country by heart and acted as our guide— there was another passenger, a young woman. Even our lunch, a test I had dreaded, went passably well. My synthetic teeth attacked the omelet, boiled fish, and cup custard with bravado, and it all slid down without resistance.

By midafternoon, thirsty but euphoric, we drove up to a spacious house surrounded by flowering terraces. It was irresistible. We were given a cordial welcome, and I was shown into a comfortable room with French doors opening onto a balcony blooming with yellow and blue pansies, and beyond it, a picture-postcard view over the mountains. My first impression blossomed into ecstasy. Having unpacked my bag and put my things away, I read the list of regulations that patients were asked to observe. The only one I could possibly have objected to involved punctuality in the dining room, and since I was to have my meals in my room, there wasn't even that to threaten the feeling of independence essential to my well-being.

Before two days were out, I had staked out my position on the margin of the establishment's communal life, and let the personnel know that punctuality and order were not among my virtues. I left my room in the morning, came back for lunch, left in the middle of the afternoon, and returned just in time for dinner. The schedule changed little, except that sometimes I came home later than other times. In the beginning, the maids tried timidly to make me respect the regulations. It was clear that we had very different ideas about these. I warned them gently that their hopes were fruitless and that they couldn't expect to succeed where so many others had failed. My wife, for instance. . . .

In due course, they accepted me for what I was: an untidy and undisciplined writer. I'm sure that in their eyes, I was a hopeless case and a disaster for any wife. Wherever I happen to be, the place becomes a wild jumble of papers, books, magazines, notes, and odd pieces of clothing. The maids finally solved the problem by leaving my meals in covered dishes in the midst of the disorder. Their love of order didn't make them any less human. Their main concern was to make sure I was comfortable and regaining my health, even if I wasn't God's gift to a convalescent home.

As I ate my meals by the open French doors and instructed my inexperienced teeth in how to perform their new function, my eyes drank in the changing light on the mountains. I would follow the progress of a cloud over the snow on a distant summit, a dull gray as the cloud's shadow passed over it, glistening white as soon as the sun reappeared. Then my eyes would dwell on the tiny chapel that someone had seen fit to build high up on a rocky ledge. Had it been placed high up there, the better to proclaim its faith to the entire valley? Faith is a beautiful thing. The faith of my childhood is always just below the surface, and I felt myself in some way protected by those stones heaped high for love of the Virgin.

On the other hand, I did miss the protection of a lock on my door. (I didn't know this was done in all convalescent homes.) I had nothing to fear, either for my fortune or for my virtue, but I wouldn't have liked to be caught trying to put together my new smile. Luckily, I was protected from unwarranted callers by a tall screen which preserved the secrets of my "toilette." To people of my generation, modesty and self-respect are closely related.

Faithful to my original intention, I made no secret of the disease that was making this splendid holiday possible. But I soon learned that it wasn't to be mentioned in this particular establishment, geared to curing everything but "that." The rule of silence, the presumption that "cancer didn't exist" was a convenience. It made it possible for me to avoid contact with the other patients as a threat to my morale. I saw them in the halls, in the library, in the lobby; I smiled and said a few words here and there, but that was all. Even on rainy afternoons, I avoided the television room and its mind-numbing entertainment; I simply bought an umbrella.

During the morning, I took my sunbath on a terrace that appeared to be the exclusive province of women. Mostly middle-aged, they sat in chairs and knitted as they gossiped. I didn't try to join in their conversation, nor did they invite me to, suggesting rather than I was an impostor in what they regarded as their preserve. My ascots may have given them the impression that I belonged to an indeterminate sex of questionable morals. Actually, I was there because there wasn't a single room available in the men's wing.

My first week in the mountains was one of exploration, discovery and, to a certain extent, recovery of the past. Along the banks of the road that led to the nearest town, the wildflowers had the colors of my youth, of my days as an eight- or nine-year-old schoolboy walking home with my brother along a narrow Normandy road. How could I have forgotten the smell of hawthorne or the sharpness of its prickers? As I rediscovered the countryside, I marveled that I could feel so clean, so new, so young—why not?—in this limpid air, conditioned only by nature. My shirt pocket stuffed with flowers, gentians, daisies, dandelions (I wasn't particular), I broached the old fortified town and its imposing gate, not as a tourist but as a neighbor. Tall houses, steep streets, dark alleys, a tiny church square, dominating ramparts, and fountains everywhere. I was still a little weak in the legs, and there was one particular step that challenged my dignity. I couldn't make it without using my hands. I was tempted to make a detour but stuck with it. Long before my month was up, the step had dwindled to nothing.

"Old stones" generally leave me unmoved. I'm much more interested in life than in three-star ancient cities, and this old town was full of it. It was June, so the place was still fresh from its snow-laden winter and making leisurely preparations for the onslaught of summer visitors. The atmosphere was relaxed and happy. There were few people in the streets, and those who were seemed always to know each other, calling out greetings, stopping to chat, exchanging hearty laughter. As for me, after an errand or two, and the attention of a few stray dogs, I stopped at a café where both owner and clients seemed glad to include me in.

They knew where I was staying, why I was there. I hid neither my profession nor my illness. A man gives his friendship to the degree that he knows where to place you. I held nothing back. As the days passed, I ventured farther into the town. My calves toughened, my skin darkened, my circle of friends widened from the charming old lady who ran a souvenir shop to the little girls erupting out of school, from the librarian to the pharmacist, from noisy students to shuffling old men. Between the old town and my room, my life was in perfect balance: on the one hand, the pleasure of new faces in a new place; on the other, the peaceful calm of my solitude. I slept well, the food tasted good, my red corpuscles were increasing. The medical staff was very pleased with me.

With such a sequence of happy days, a month goes by very fast. It was a memorable time for me, beyond anything I ever expected. A state of grace? Perhaps. Of egotism? Absolutely.

July and its holiday crowds broke the charm. The air became heavier. Canned music blared through the narrow streets, insulting the past, the past the inhabitants were trying to sell. The "season" was on, and I was leaving just in time not to sully the image I was taking home. I made my farewells, and early the next morning, after a last look at the tiny chapel high on its rock, I took the road back to Paris. Happily, it was the same driver. However, this time he was in a great hurry. The trip home from a holiday is seldom enjoyable.

I surprised my family at their lunch. They had not expected me so early, though they should be surprised at nothing. My wife immediately observed that, in spite of my tan, I looked tired. Nothing escapes that woman. . . . To be sure, the trip had been hurried, with only two brief stops, one for the vehicle, one for the passengers. She also noticed—which she didn't tell me until much later when it had subsided—that my face had taken on an odd shape. My chin had become square—shades of Popeye!—and my lower jaw was strangely swollen around the edge of the radiated zone. I knew I felt pain in that area, but when I looked at myself in the mirror with fond and understandable indulgence, the transformation had somehow escaped me. Love is blind; I must love myself more than I know.

I timidly brought the matter up with my doctors, but they seemed little concerned. They were interested in efficacy, not aesthetics. When a doctor tells you "you look great," take it with a grain of salt. He sees only your case; that's his job and he's right. Better to look like a live Popeye than a beautiful corpse.

4

The next morning, well rested and as cheerful as the day was beautiful, I set forth on trembling legs to show off my burnished face to the dwindling neighborhood. Some of the shops had already closed for summer vacation, and those children who hadn't been provided with a holiday in the country took over the sidewalks with the noisy license of small Paris prisoners.

"So, you're back! You certainly look much better." Things became complicated when I had to admit: "Yes, I would have liked to stay longer, but I have to start new treatments today."

"New treatments?"

"Yes. Chemotherapy."

Chemotherapy! The word sounded like something out of science fiction. I had familiarized myself with it, tamed it as I had its forerunners, in order to use it easily and to reduce its menace. But despite my research in dictionaries and the indications I had been given by my hematologist, the treatment remained very nebulous in my mind. All I knew was that I was to appear once a

[84]

week for a month, then every ten days for the following month, to have a blood count taken, with special attention to the white count, before I was injected with five different chemicals with barbarous names and very high costs. The price is designed to instill confidence in the patient: the more expensive the medication, the better he feels. I felt almost proud to be the beneficiary of a free treatment born of the most recent scientific discoveries. The era of the mouse-fairy or guinea pig behind me, I was now spear-heading the advance into unknown territory, armed with the delusion that my case was more interesting than most, and might even be exceptional.

Early in the afternoon, my wife and I set off for the private clinic where I was to have my treatments. Since the two public hospitals with facilities for chemotherapy were overburdened and inconvenient for me, my doctor had chosen a highly respected private institution at the same price. A clinic for the very rich, a clinic for very important people, yet another reason for feeling flattered, and lucky.

"How do you feel?" the doctor asked, after carefully injecting me with the repertoire of medications prescribed by his colleague.

"Just fine, thank you, Doctor," I said, with the self-satisfied smirk of a man who is afraid of nothing.

That is not the way I felt, however, when I was stretched out on an outsized ironing board and hooked up to a bottle of glucose hanging from a metal tree. It's a very odd sensation to watch the gyrating bubbles as a liquid slowly empties into your veins, and the technician reels off the names of the beneficial poisons in the syringes she hands to the doctor.

What is it going to do to me? What do I feel? Scared, that's what I felt. An instinctive animal fear I couldn't suppress. Could the doctor guess what was going on in my head? I doubt it. He wasn't there to imagine things but to do his job.

"I didn't feel a thing," I said to the technician.

"But be careful you don't get tired, now," she said, wisely passing over any mention of the small inconveniences that chemotherapy was likely to cause. Of course, no two people react the same way.

Feeling no effects, I returned home, complimenting myself on my robust constitution, and picked up my activities where I had left off.

The Fourteenth of July arrived, with its republican fireworks and parade of soldiers, increasingly motorized, and reinforced by a female contingent marching with measured steps, demonstrating that women were no longer just the warrior's rest and recreation. Radio and television commentators added their virile tones to the patriotic tremolo of the military bands, swelling the epic pageantry of the glorious occasion. There was almost the same passion used to describe football games. The past always forgotten, the crowds applauded the spanking new army they had paid for out of their own pockets, and the solemn figures in the official stands patted each other on the back. Vanity and illusion!

The next Monday came all too soon. The second session was no different from the first. The white corpuscles were going down, but were still numerous enough to require the full dosage. The same panic behind my tempered smile, the same relief on finding myself safe and sound after what seemed an eternity. "Good-bye. Thank you. See you next Monday."

This time, I was much less brisk on my walk home. I was beginning to suspect that "Paris in August," the season so dear to writers, was going to be no bed of roses. In fact, I would be spending it on a bed of much more modest periwinkle. The base of one of my medications was indeed periwinkle. They were feeding my blood periwinkle! What a pleasant thought! A flower can't be evil; it's innocent.

By the end of July, most of Paris had disappeared. By imitation, perhaps, so had a large number of my corpuscles of both colors. I wasn't to worry, it was anticipated in the program. Corpuscles are capricious; they come and go.

One evening, my wife told me she had been talking about my case with a friend.

"He told me that after three and a half years, it couldn't be the same cancer they operated on the first time."

"Really? You mean I had a new one?"

"Yes, and that makes it much less serious. It's cured faster."

Two small cancers instead of one big one! Her good intentions were laudable, but still, two cancers to one man seemed excessive. True, the rich get richer. When I repeated her remark to my hematologist, he gave me a dirty look and barked: "Who told you that?" I stammered that my wife had, and that she had done so out of pure love.

August came to an end. The summer exodus was over; traffic was once more bumper-to-bumper. On the other hand, my red corpuscles did not return. To replace them, I played host to some from my blood group. Gorged with these new transfusions, I could look forward to two weeks between sessions. A few unpleasant hours every other week were tolerable enough.

"Your nausea reactions are the same as a woman's in

the early stages of pregnancy," was the technician's comment when I ventured to tell her about my symptoms. As soon as she had put a Band-Aid on the perforated vein, I quickly dressed and jumped into one of the taxis that always seemed to be ready and waiting outside the clinic door. (It was a good taxi stand; the clinic had a well-heeled clientele.) But oh, that trip home! The interminable crawl along the boulevard saturated with cars often at a standstill, with my soul in torment and my heart in my mouth. I had the terrible sensation that I was a sick and impotent prisoner caught in a tide of roaring, stink-exuding metal, more alone and abandoned than in the most impenetrable jungle or deserted desert. The sensation of being about to die without anyone raising a finger to save me; the certainty that I would breathe my last without anyone being any the wiser. A half-hour's trip on good days; more often a whole hour; one night during a transportation strike, two hours. Then the effort to pay the driver, thank him in the fewest possible words, and fling myself into the elevator—thank God it was working!—and finally reach my door before the end came. Once the nausea was behind me, I stretched out in a state of exhaustion; finally to sleep, then to wake up two or three hours later, wiggle one arm, wiggle the other, and realize that I was still among the living. The relief was indescribable.

September, October, life ran its course. Each month I saw the surgeon and the radiologist at the hospital. For the time being, all was well. As for the future, they were silent. Not all doctors believe in chemotherapy. Physically, I left much to be desired, but my morale was holding up.

Not my wife's. She was always coming home with

contradictory opinions about my treatments. The day before one of my perfusions, knowing how I dreaded the next day, my wife could no longer hold back her anxiety over my slow recovery and suggested I stop the treatments. She knew as well as I that a cure in the fullest sense of the word was out of the question. The doctor had committed himself only to a remission, obviously with no idea about its duration.

Since every living person is in a state of remission from the moment he is born, the word is not especially alarming. Given my functional optimism, it allowed me to contemplate a serene old age. Why not? The moment, or whatever we think of as temporary, is usually what lasts longest.

"What if you didn't go?" she asked. "What if you stopped the perfusions?"

Although I knew that she was motivated solely by affection, I expressed my gratitude in an explosion of deliberately exaggerated rage. Because I had been wondering too. For all my confidence and determination to stay the course, I questioned the effectiveness of the treatments, especially with another one facing me the next day. I was sorely tempted to throw in the towel, to turn coward. I had to be nasty, even use ugly language, to bolster my wavering resolve.

When I'd calmed down, I said: "Chemotherapy is a very difficult treatment. But I'm damned lucky to have it." Thus I placed myself among the privileged few.

November was not a good month. For one thing, my lower jaw had contracted, and, as a result, my temporary denture had a tendency to wander around. Sometimes I could eat fairly normally; other times I felt as if my mouth were full of dice.

Even more important, and a source of greater anxiety,

I was having more and more trouble conjugating the verb "to love." I lacked the desire; I lacked the means. I had read enough to know that chemotherapy often caused this type of deficiency, but I had somehow hoped I'd be spared. It didn't obsess me, but I certainly didn't like the idea of doing without. At a time when sex is king and available almost everywhere, it seemed unfortunate to be deprived of it. I wanted to feel capable of responding to provocation—without that, what's the use of dreaming?—and I felt ashamed to seem deaf and dumb at its approach. What kind of writer are you if you can't make love? Was I Abelard to a new generation of Héloïses?

In line with the old morality so dear to doctors, that their patients should know as little as possible about what ails them, my doctor had been very conscientious about listing the side effects of interest to him, but not those that interested me. When I saw him at the end of the month, I was not feeling at all well disposed.

"I've been giving you the drastic treatment," he said. Then, looking at me out of the corner of his eye, "And you haven't taken it very well."

No need to say more: my wife must have telephoned him without telling me.

I became more specific.

"Doctor," I said, "I haven't smoked for four years, I don't drink anymore, and if at this point I can't . . ."—out of politeness, I replaced the verb with an equally explicit pause—"what do I have left? Of course I want a remission, but not just any old remission. If my life is going to be cut out from under me, I don't want it."

"You'll be all right," he reassured me. "The worst is behind you. Everything will be as it was."

"I insist upon it, Doctor."

He examined me at length and cut my perfusions down to one a month, using a "cocktail" (that's the word he used) in which he would replace the medication I had had particular difficulty tolerating with something to control the nausea, plus a prescription to restore my prowess as a functioning male. I wouldn't be seeing him for another six months, but I could always call him in case of need. But he was sure everything would be all right. It was.

Day by day, week by week, I regained my vitality, and with it, the delight of putting it to good use.

By mid-December, I had begun to gain weight and was looking more presentable. I could see it reflected in people's faces. Even if you weren't completely cured of cancer, you could still learn to live with it. The people in my neighborhood who had been so eager to bury me were duly impressed. So that they wouldn't seem to have been mistaken—people don't like admitting mistakes— they attributed my restored health to an unusually strong constitution and a willpower bordering on the miraculous.

Miraculous is a big word, but my attitude toward my disease was closely linked to the way my system functioned. A man is all of a piece. The young man who, four years earlier, had said, "If I had cancer, I'd put a bullet through my head," told me one evening: "Now that I know you better, now that I've seen you. . . . Well, if I had cancer now, I'd do exactly what you've done."

Now, I've never intended or pretended to be an example to anyone. I do battle for my own benefit, I am an egotist. But still, the thought that I could influence a young man to be less pessimistic about cancer was very gratifying. What I had done, the way I had acted, could be useful to other people. Not to all, unfortunately, for you first have to find the courage inside yourself. And you have to be lucky. . . .

This new role as a man of public usefulness had repercussions. People questioned me, asked my advice: they had a parent, a friend. . . . I confined my words of wisdom to: "I had it treated, I am still having it treated, and here I am." Then, to undo all my good work, came the headline one gray December day: "Doctor Lacassagne, cancer specialist, committed suicide when he learned he had been stricken with the disease." I was horrified. There it was, in black and white. So that no one could miss it. Despicable! What about the others? All those with cancer across the length and breadth of the land? What hope would they have after such an act? And he an expert! Should they all commit suicide too?

I was furious with the newspapers for printing this poison to jack up their sales without considering for a minute the harm they were doing. After all, people with cancer can still read. To make matters worse, the two reporters assigned to the story—not one but two!—had the gall to write: "Doctor Antoine Lacassagne, Director of the Institut Curie, chose an exemplary death!" An old man of eighty-seven, his breakfast eaten, had thrown himself out of his sixth-story window. They call that an exemplary death! Then, in a few oily lines, they tried to justify the lamentable end of a man of great probity who was experiencing perhaps his first and certainly his last defeat. Besides, for me there isn't this or that kind of death. There is death, and that's it. What follows? . . .

Sickened by such a show of mischievous stupidity, I expressed my indignation to all who would listen. But for each person who was as revolted as I was, there were many more who didn't understand my position at all. He had cancer and committed suicide. So what? What was so unusual about it? Wasn't it logical? Cancer is the worst of all diseases, an incurable disease as everyone knows. The best proof was this doctor's act. He knew it!

I would try to defend my point of view, underscoring the cruelty of that story to other cancer victims. People listened politely. "Ah, yes, of course. It isn't good for those poor people, is it? Not good at all. You're quite right." But they lacked conviction and were eager to change the conversation. Cancer is so frightening that no one wants to talk about it, except when it's a question of the great scientific strides being made against "the scourge," each person thinking: "Cancer will be beaten before I get it!" As for those with cancer now, they are pitied, of course, but nothing can be done about them; they are under sentence of death, so it's best to forget them.

That same evening, still full of indignation, I reluctantly bought two more copies of the paper and carefully cut out the offending story. Then, my anger at the boil, I took up my pen and wrote two almost identical letters, one to a left-wing paper, the other to an extreme right-wing sheet, asking them to give space to the protestations of a man unfortuanately well placed—I forced that one a bit—to combat the particularly odious tone of the enclosed article. Pleased with my efforts, I dropped the letters in the mailbox . . . and waited. Two months later, the right-wing paper wrote me a very friendly and full replay that smacked of a letter of condolence. But neither paper had seen fit to publish my letter in their readers' column.

They knew their business. Only scandals that arouse a large public outcry, and maintain, or better still, increase, a newspaper's circulation are given an airing.

Cancer is sometimes a good subject; the cancer patient, never. If, for example, an organization or individual uses its profits to aid research in new weapons to fight the disease, that's a good thing. To the man on the street, his pocketbook and his health are very sensitive subjects, and he is always on the side of those working for the good of the public, meaning him. He may swear he won't give another cent, then that well-known face—it must be a friend since he looks so familiar—addresses him from the television screen, face oozing compassion, voice suitably unctuous, and makes yet another appeal to his generosity. Abusing a person's trust is not necessarily a sin; naiveté is made to be exploited. I'm not against charity, only against the insidious way it is manipulated in the name of progress. What horrors are perpetrated in the name of progress! With expectable regularity, you're asked to succor the indigent, the blind, the handicapped, those sticken with polio, the aged, the starving throughout the world. They're after you to support research here, to set up a foundation there, to protect endangered species or stray dogs, and each time, men of goodwill give. But for a neighbor with cancer? Not a chance! Cancer in general is one thing; a person with cancer quite another.

Looking back, I now see how ill-timed and foolish my protestation was. How they must have laughed in those newspaper offices! A man with cancer complaining about his lot. What next! People who theoretically already belonged to the past should realize that their opinions are of little interest to a world they will soon be leaving. In the process, they managed to discourage those less stubborn than I. I took comfort in a proverb, Arab, I think, that goes something like this: "If a man should do you harm, don't be angry. Instead, go sit by the side of a river and watch the eddies in the current. By and by, you will see your enemy's corpse float by."

My fruitless involvement with the press behind me, I resumed my hazardous course through the small daily pleasures, the larger hopes for the future, and the financial woes that are the price of personal freedom. Christmas was upon us, and a few days before, I noticed that my hair was falling out at an alarming rate. Apparently there is no such thing as undiluted happiness. I knew, though not from my doctor who was above such minor considerations, that loss of hair was yet another result of chemotherapy, but I had depended on my heretofore impervious head of hair to protect me from this new aesthetic affront. I knew from my prisoner-of-war experience that baldness did not become me. My scalp is covered with bumps and my ears are too big. Some woman is sure to tell you: "A man can be bald and desirable at the same time. Look at Yul Brynner!" It varies according to age, cultures, tastes, but it's my impression that such handsome and hairless seducers are mostly found in novels written by authors whose youth is well behind them.

Trying to make it with a pretty girl while wearing a toupee and a denture is bound to end in humiliating defeat. Short of paying for it, of course, which negates the argument. It's true that I don't understand women, or so my wife tells me, but so much the better, since it gives me reason to hope. No man wants to believe that his days of amorous conquests are over. Even for a happily married man, the desire to be attractive to women is not considered a sin, nor does it have a statute of limitations.

While a dental prosthesis seemed more of a nuisance

than a handicap, I felt I was too old to hide my scalp under the exotic headgear of a hippie or pseudo-artist. I don't mind being laughed at, but I want to be the one to decide the moment. When I questioned my doctor about my vanishing hair, he said: "Don't give it a thought! Your hair will grow back in no time, and it will be more luxuriant than ever. Everybody who's been treated with periwinkle knows that."

As I've said before, my experience with doctors, in whom I otherwise have the greatest faith, has taught me to be very suspicious where minor—to them—side effects are concerned. They are consummate liars. Even though my hematologist is much younger than I, his hairline is already receding well up his forehead. In his case, it suits his calling well, and his patients regard it as a reassuring sign of experience and seriousness. Those two words give me pause. In my case, experience has taught me nothing, and I equate seriousness with being bored.

My wife was very sympathetic. She shared my anxiety and was beginning to think the fates were overdoing it. With a sure instinct for which I am continually grateful, she found a new product derived from a plant base that smelled of eucalyptus. By rubbing it regularly into my scalp, I had a gleaming mane in no time. If I had to choose between my doctor's "I told you so" and my bottle of heady ointment, I'd give full marks to the latter. Moreover, where before I had begun to go gray—lacking other riches, a little silver at the temples is not a bad substitute—my hair had now returned to its youthful chestnut.

There is an old French saying: "A fool's hair never turns white." Am I a fool? Who's to say? You're always a fool to someone or about someone. In any event, I started the new year with zest and a new set of ascots for my neck. My wife has excellent taste in ascots and they received many a compliment, mostly from women. And since ties are being worn less and less, I felt entirely with it. Carrying a sentence of "ascots for life," I could only hope that fashions didn't change too soon—in the garment trade, they're capable of anything—and that the shirt of our fathers with the obligatory closing at the neck never returned.

To cap the Christmas largesse, I had my first perfusion of the new year when it was only three days old. And even though the new "cocktail" was effective against the nauseous side effects, I was still in agony before, during, and after the ordeal. Then, in the middle of that first week, I had an experience that still makes me wince. I was going out to buy my newspaper when my son asked me if I'd pick up a certain periodical for him. After taking my faithful *Canard* from the pile, I asked the young news vendor for my son's publication. My temporary choppers (the permanent ones were still in the works) had begun to take on a life of their own, and I guess my pronunciation left something to be desired.

"You want what?" he said.

I repeated my request with infinite care, but the young man said "What?" again, this time laughing lustily. Thinking I was doing it as a joke, he wanted to join in the fun. "You shouldn't talk with your mouth full," he said with a wink.

I wanted to throttle him. In a rage, I muttered a clearly understandable "That's enough, now; I don't like to be made fun of," found the magazine, yanked it off the rack, paid for it, and turned on my heels. The poor boy stood stunned and speechless at my exhibition of bad humor, whose origin he couldn't possibly understand.

I continued to buy my papers from him, but I didn't speak to him for a long time. Pick up paper; put down money. Vexation does not become a man. Once I had my new teeth, I let drop on occasional word. Now we're on the best of terms, and I gossip with him for minutes on end. I was wrong on every count. I should have laughed with him, but above all, I shouldn't have carried my grudge for such a long time. The young man certainly didn't deserve it. And in my case, it became a bore and a nuisance because I couldn't figure out how to bring it to an end without losing face. It's one of the few experiences from which I've learned something.

What I've learned is to take the bull by the horns. When I'm about to have a conversation with someone I don't know, I try to put him, but mostly me, at ease by saying: "I'm sorry if I don't always speak clearly, but I've just had an operation and I have to wear this gadget that I'm still not used to," following this with a vague gesture toward my mouth and a winning smile. Both of us are spared. My interlocutor then says: "I have no trouble understanding you," or "It isn't noticeable at all," and I can splutter with impunity. The one hazard that dogs me is my overabundant saliva; when it's misplaced, even the most indulgent are put off.

January, February, and March went well. My weight shot up with the price of meat and was nearing the ideal. Ideal perhaps, but in my precarious financial condition, it created a serious wardrobe problem. In midwinter, with our climate, an ascot is not enough. And flapping like a scarecrow in last winter's clothes might confirm my friends' worst fears. "He's had it, all right. He's done for."

When you're wearing a jacket much too large for you,

how can you convince anyone that you're really trying to gain weight? The opposite, yes, and with what ill-concealed pleasure! Kindness does not come naturally in "civilized" countries, but worse still, it puts ideas in your head. Wearing clothes that are too large diminishes the man inside them. It promotes an inferiority complex. And although I had no wish to regain all the superfluous pounds sacrificed to my recuperation, I did want a few back. They had been my reserve; without them, what would have become of me? But at what point would my weight be stabilized? I couldn't take the risk of ordering new suits which I might not be able to wear. (The good old days when tailors "forgot" to present their bills to favored customers are long since gone. Too bad. Manners also are a thing of the past.) I therefore adopted the economical recourse of sweaters. They gave me the casual look I associated with artists, and they had the great virtue of elasticity. Fat or lean, I was covered.

Spring arrived and so did the lilies of the valley. I'm not referring to the ones that blossom punctually on May Day in Paris flower shops, but to those which insidiously rushed the season and established themselves in my mouth. My mucous membrane was covered with little white dots. Naturally I rushed to my doctor and asked him what these horrors—not unusual in an infant but totally unsuitable to a man my age—were doing in my mouth.

It was always impossible to guess what he was thinking. Not much that was cheerful, was my guess. He spoke little, as I've already mentioned, and neither his words nor the expression on his face gave me an inkling of what was going on in his mind.

"You are still having chemotherapy?" he asked me,

after examining me and giving me a prescription for an antibiotic.

"Yes, Doctor."

He looked annoyed, perhaps even a little worried.

"You must stop it immediately. I'll write a note to your doctor right away."

I couldn't have hoped for anything nicer than an end to the chemotherapy. I knew that there were risks in the treatment and that my natural defense mechanism would be taking a beating. My flowering mouth was a sign of vulnerability. I'd already surmised that this doctor wasn't sold on chemotherapy, for all its beneficial results. I was also fairly certain that my hematologist would take an opposing view, but the final say would rest with the senior faculty, so it was out of my hands. Coward that I am, I seized the opportunity to cancel the next perfusion and advanced the date for the tests and examination scheduled for the end of my course of treatments. One perfusion less was no small victory. With my mouth returned to normal, I took heart and threw myself into preparations for my nephew's impending marriage.

It was with little enthusiasm that I went two weeks later to see my hematologist. It took no crystal ball to guess that he would be displeased, and I regretted that I would be an unintentional source of irritation to a man already overburdened with work and worry.

As I expected, his greeting was less than cordial.

"What do you mean, dropping your treatments when you were nearly eighty percent done?" he snapped.

"It wasn't my idea. My surgeon said I should stop them. He said he was writing you to that effect."

"It's not for him to say when to stop them. That's my job."

After listing the various arguments for continuing

treatments that were obviously showing good results, he shot out:

"All right. You decide!"

Startled, I replied with some heat:

"Doctor, as you are well aware, I have complete confidence in you, just as I have in my surgeon. Don't ask me to choose between you. I can't do it. If I obey him and put an end to the chemotherapy, you'll say: 'Since you're not doing what I told you to do, there is no point in your coming to see me.' If, on the other hand, I continue your treatment, he'll be angry and lose all interest in a patient who refuses to follow his advice. Either way, I lose. Now, when I was told, not once but twice, 'You must have an operation and as soon as possible,' I said yes, although I could have refused. With your advice, I took full responsibility for my decision. Today, I can't do it. For several years now I've entrusted the problem of my health to the two of you, and it's up to you together to sort out my future and decide what is best for me."

A doctor's lot is not an easy one, and there are times when, morally speaking, the patient's position is less difficult than the doctor's. He has to decide another man's fate and make decisions on the basis of what he knows and what his conscience tells him. It's no joking matter. We discussed the problem a little further, enough to come to an understanding. It's a rare doctor who is willing to argue with a patient. Yet there are patients who need to be told at least something. Of course there are limits. . . .

There was a moment of silence. The doctor seemed to be turning things over in his mind as he darted a quizzical look at me through his glasses. Then suddenly his face lit up and he gave me a big smile, the wide youthful smile of a man who has licked a problem.

"Okay, I'll write to him," he said, and asked me to get undressed. He was pleased with my physical condition, prescribed a much-reduced treatment for the next eight months, the monthly perfusions continuing but the dose reduced to two easily tolerated elements, one of them the indispensable periwinkle.

With the heavy infusion of spinach provided by my dear wife, I began to swell like a toad. Shades of Popeye! But at least my jaw had returned to normal and my new teeth were gradually becoming personalized. The spring sun added a touch of color to my face, clients for my wares appeared in increasing numbers, and I was the very personification of hope.

During the course of the spring, I talked a few neighbors into having themselves looked over at the hospital where I still went for periodic examinations. Among them were smokers, "moderate" drinkers, some persistent coughers. Because it was a simple precaution, they were less apprehensive about the results. A cancer caught in time is curable. Wasn't I the living proof? They all came back with clean bills of health, and seemed very grateful. Having said this much, I want to make it clear that I had no intention of proselytizing inveterate smokers and drinkers. Everyone is free to do as he chooses, and, God knows, many of them were a lot healthier than I was.

Generally pleased with myself, satisfaction with self seldom forsaking me, I was ready to risk going to restaurants. Chinese were the best, for the food is virtually premasticated. Gradually I was able to extend my gastronomic forays, physically if not financially. My speech improved to the point where I didn't have to repeat myself like a parrot, and laughing was no longer a threat to my companions.

Another reason for rejoicing was that as spring returned, so did my virility. I no longer had to avoid X-rated movies. I am not made of stone and I do love movies, which doesn't mean that I'm a lover of porn. But now that the masterminds of the cinema are determined to show our children that modesty is an infirmity, masturbation a healthy occupation, and pederasty a mark of intelligence and a guarantee of upward mobility, I didn't want to be caught lagging behind the poor slobs who think that admiring sexual audacity is a sign of superior evolution. The traffickers in the pill and "erotico-medical" literature keep aiming lower, always lower. And yet, breasts and more breasts, buttocks piled on buttocks eventually depress a man's spirits, and may in turn breed impotence. Happily, sex isn't all there is to life, or love.

In June, I had to get a new passport. My old one had expired the month before, and I didn't want to find myself unable to cross the border because I lacked a rudimentary document. I had traveled very little in the last few years, but this didn't prevent me from dreaming of trips I might make in the future. Why not? An unforeseen opportunity, a lucky break, an unexpected windfall. . . . Nothing must stand in its way.

The year before, near the end of my stay in the mountains, thanks to that "Open Sesame" the French government grants to all its citizens, and a bus ticket purchased at modest cost, I had spent a day in Italy. Another happy memory! I fled the program included in the trip, herded visits to historical monuments (I detest looking for the sake of having seen; I cannot admire on command), and went off by myself on a voyage of discovery, a few thousand liras in my pocket, a dozen words I believed approximated Italian, and a desire to strike up acquaint-ances in a new land. It's a wonderful feeling to set forth on an adventure without a guide and with no aim but to take part in the daily lives of other people. What I found is not on picture postcards: my vision is made up of ar-cades, a little vermouth, sunny plazas, pretty girls who smiled at my accent, and a good meal in a place where I was the only Frenchman—spaghetti and ice cream go very well together and are easy to eat—a few statues and handsome buildings vaguely seen and soon forgotten, and many, many people who were ready to respond to my friendship with their own. My traveling companions recrossed the border, gratified that they now "knew Italy," and weighed down with ill-disguised bottles of apéritifs which testified to their having been abroad. I had only a few trinkets for the family in my pockets, and a rich harvest of impressions I savor to this day.

The photograph on my new passport was of the usual rogue's gallery variety; it's what you get with cut-rate photography. But I felt better when I noticed that the line "physical peculiarities" had been left a blank. Thanks to the speed of the sitting, my ascot had stayed in place and so the scars and tattoos on my raddled neck had not been exposed. Best of all, the passport bore in bold letters the legend: "Good for ten years from date of issue."

This statement spoke volumes: in ten years, I would have to renew the document. There are moments when I'm very respectful of the government; I promised myself to obey this injunction to the letter. I was enlisted in the army of the living for another ten years! It was as good as a guarantee. Orders from the Paris Préfecture de Police are not to be taken lightly.

5

With my July perfusion behind me, I left for my native
province, a trip I had to do without the summer before.
The countryside, my house, my fig tree, my bicycle—
nothing had changed. I picked up where I'd left off two
years earlier. In a few days, sea and sun gave me a tan,
and I left off the ascots, wearing them only for dress occasions. My scars seemed to have disappeared, or at least
I was encouraged to think so. One day on the beach, I
explained to a friend that the scars pulled if I stayed in
the water too long. Registering surprise, she said:

"What scars?"

I admit the lady was no longer young, but on the other
hand, she was not an old crone. I could even compete,
up to a point, with the young gladiators on the beach
whose thickening midsections bespoke more eating and
drinking than exercise. In some ways, cancer is a preser-
vative.

I know that my village has mixed feelings about me.
Some don't like me, some are glad to see me again, but
almost all of them view me as a curious phenomenon.

My profession, coupled with my jokes, sometimes in doubtful taste, place me somewhere between an artist and a nut. Literature having so far failed to give me the exterior signs of opulence, and the devastations of my operations and treatments not helping, the latter opinion tends to dominate.

I had no wish to correct this impression. Their appetite for life and mine were different and differently expessed. Maybe out of false pride, certainly from personal necessity, I was more active and more eccentric than ever before. It was my way of convincing myself that I was alive and well. Rain or shine, cold or windy, I swam every day according to the tides. (The tide table is the only one I ever respected.) When I wasn't over my head in water, I was astride my faithful two-wheeler, indifferent to the smiles I provoked. In contrast to the summer crowd strutting about in their resort clothes, I knew I looked like a fool and didn't give a damn.

"You're still riding that bike," a friend remarked. "The damn thing is indestructible!"

I laughed and thought how like my bike I was. Euphoric and unregenerate in my contempt for the law, I pedaled down one-way streets the wrong way, but always keeping a sharp eye out for the policeman's distinctive silhouette. Our summer police force is not only very small but very good-natured. The risks were small.

My old friends didn't know what to make of me. We had chosen different roads. Most of them were heading toward mandatory retirement, paid for through the nose, while I had chosen a life of improvisation without end, like a schoolboy. And when my one remaining and much-loved aunt had occasion to scold me, I accepted it with the humility of a guilty child. It's not such a bad thing to be scolded from time to time.

Even if unrecognized as a medical fact, salt air leads to thirst, and my little peninsula, surrounded on three sides at high tide, was well provided with cafés, bistros, and bars of all sizes. The owner of one of them was an old friend, and I often stopped by for a chat. At the apéritif hour, I knew almost his entire clientele, and I'd known his one and only waiter since he was a child. He still addressed me as "sir," whereas the rest of the crowd called me either by my first name or "the barefoot boy." (It happens that I get very attached to a pair of espa- drilles and wear them until I'm literally walking on the soles of my own feet. I like the sensation. Instead of get- ting worn, my own soles thicken as the summer progres- ses. We call it "walking pilgrim-style.")

One morning I was there earlier than usual. I noticed that my old friend was constantly clearing his throat as he talked. Something was obviously bothering him. I couldn't help asking if something was wrong with his throat.

"Oh, it's just a small irritation," he said.

"Have you seen anybody about it?"

"Sure, I went to see a doctor, a specialist, but he didn't find anything."

I said no more. I didn't want him to think that just because I'd had a cancer in the same region, it gave me the right to consign one to him. But, putting together his age, his chain-smoking, and his line of work, and now this nasty persistent little cough, I had to place him among the strong contenders, if not an out-and-out win- ner.

Near the middle of August, I had to make a quick trip to Paris. Seven hundred and fifty miles so as not to miss a perfusion is proof of a clear conscience. On my return, the groups on the beach had thinned out. The sunsets were more beautiful. Then came September. Since we were among the lucky mortals with a second home—shared with termites, to be sure—and with my profession, such as it was, I could put off the dread return to Paris, dreaded ever since return meant "back to school."

With summer come to an end, September was, as in most summer resorts, the month for weddings among the local young. The weather was still beautiful, work had slackened off, and in my view, autumn has it all over spring for making love. My friend's café was opposite the town hall, the church was close by, and the procession usually went on foot from the bureaucracy's seals and stamps to the priest's benediction. Then came the feast, and later . . . ah, later!

My friend was as husky and healthy as ever, but he still had his cough. It annoyed me because, for all his denials, it was clear that his "little thing" was beginning to bother him too. I had been down that road, and the thoughts I had had then must be much like the ones he was having now. "Little things" that won't go away arouse an instinctive suspicion that reason shouldn't be allowed to combat. "Little things" are to be closely watched. "Suspicion is the mother of security," the poet said. People should listen to poets more often. It wouldn't be easy to warn my friend without alarming him, nor to suggest that no matter how competent his doctor, this disease cannot be diagnosed at a preliminary examination. And yet to hold my tongue was hard too.

What to do? I hit on the cowardly solution of telling his wife—after all, everybody knew he was a stubborn brute—and advised her to send her husband back to the specialist, the sooner the better. Before returning to Paris, I tried to share my optimism with my friend, treating cancer not as something likable (I'm not that far gone yet) but at least as something this side of cata-strophic and not always deserving of its bad reputation.

During the course of the summer, I discussed the question of life insurance with an old friend, but he wasn't very hopeful. "You can always try," he said with a weak smile, "But it would surprise me." There was a paradox here that disturbed me. On the one hand, the law was using every form of coercion at its command to force me to provide for my retirement, while on the other, I was refused any kind of life insurance. My instinct for logic and justice was outraged. Having as always no money to spend either on my retirement or on a life insurance policy, I put off for the moment my desire to plumb the mystery behind these opposing views of my longevity.

Came the day when we turned off the meters, locked the doors, and headed back to Paris. As soon as we reached the Loire, the weather turned dismal, confirming the weather forecasters who always attribute to this stately river the character of a rigid barrier between good weather and bad. Heading north and toward what was awaiting me, I didn't need forecasts to tell me I was returning to a cloudy future.

For two months I had kept my worries at bay; now they were lying in wait to repossess me. As we ticked off the miles, I tried to reduce them to manageable proportions: I had this on the fire, another project looked good. If my sanguine disposition has taught me nothing else, it is that a financial hemorrhage isn't fatal so long as you have your health. By the time we reached the outskirts of Paris, my passing pessimism had evaporated. It wasn't a return but a beginning. I would enter the fray with renewed vigor, determined to triumph.

By October, my incorrigible optimism was proving justified. A television play I had written and been paid for three years earlier and assumed to be forgotten, suddenly emerged from the depths and was awaiting filming. A young cameraman and I set off for Alsace in search of a location resembling Poland (my story involved a tender memory of that land). The choice wasn't as odd as it sounds. Pine trees are pine trees, barracks from the last war—the *last* war, this I swear—usually have the same Germanic outline, and the snow covering the characters would obliterate their nationality.

We knew we could depend on snow and we had more pines than we needed, but the only barracks we could find were a memorial to war atrocities, not a good background for a love story. We returned to Paris officially frustrated in our quest, although I personally relished the autumn sunshine in a part of France I barely knew. One Sunday, I had even crossed the Rhine for a cup of coffee, partly for the pleasure of using my new passport at the border, partly to send postcards to various friends, writing the inevitable banalities, not so much to tell them I was thinking of them as to demonstrate that I must be in rugged health since I was "abroad." The stamp counts for more than the distance traveled, and Frenchmen have no idea of geography anyway.

One night near the end of October, I received a telephone call from the wife of my friend, the café owner, confirming what I'd feared. He did indeed have cancer of the throat, and she wanted me to make an appointment for him with my doctor as soon as possible. He would be arriving the next day.

"We are all stricken," she said.

I knew the town well enough to imagine how the

neighbors would be carrying on. In the provinces, things must be done in a certain way or you risk general disapproval. A windfall, a piece of good luck is hushed up; people might be envious. On the other hand, a misfortune must be shared with everybody, otherwise you do them out of the opportunity of showing their sympathy and compassion.

I could visualize the scene all too clearly. "Cancer! How awful!" And they'd trot out all the words designed to keep the pain fresh and deepen a despair already made black by the word itself. And my friend's profession being what it was, with his café open winter as well as summer, he had dozens of friends who must be streaming through the house all day. I bet they spared him little.

His wife went on to explain that her husband would be staying with one or another of their three grown children who lived near Paris while he was undergoing treatment. I was able to get an appointment for him for two days later, and felt a certain pride in knowing that it was my attitude toward cancer that had helped him face his. Then I had second thoughts: What if things turned out badly for him: Wouldn't his family place the blame on me? I would have recommended the wrong doctor, hence the wrong treatment, etc., etc. I knew it was risky, if not downright dangerous, to take responsibility for someone else's illness. So I called my friend's oldest son and explained my doubts. He put my mind at rest. As soon as his father arrived, I went over to see him, playing the role of the old veteran, survivor of many battles, come to give a reassuring pat on the back to the young recruit about to go over the top. I explained, I joked, I minimized. I think my visit, and the frequent telephone calls while he was undergoing treatment, may have given him that little extra measure of confidence that his family, for all its deep affection, could not.

A few weeks later, my current series of perfusions was finished. I went to my hematologist with a secret and very wan hope that in view of my brimming health, further perfusions would be unnecessary, or could at least be spaced out. I had tried with diabolical finesse to worm some word about my perfusions out of the technicians, but they were always on their guard. They smiled and laughed and chatted about this and that, but on that subject they were suddenly deaf and dumb. "It depends on the patient. . . . It's for the doctor to decide. . . . See you next month."

They were cleverer than I, and faithfully observed one of the golden rules of their profession: be very careful with patients who are too eager to learn the truth. Just as with the doctors: you must have faith, and blind faith is preferable.

"No, I won't fill out this questionnaire."

"Why not, Doctor?"

"Professional secrets."

"But since I know what I have, or very nearly"—you must never seem too knowing—"what possible difference can it make?"

"I have no intention of giving an insurance company information about you."

A little put out, I reclaimed the detailed, not to say indiscreet, questionnaire which a highly skeptical insurance agent had given me. My experiment to see if a cancer victim could get life insurance seemed to be running into trouble. That a doctor should refuse to state in black and white that I'd had two operations for cancer, that much I could understand. So I tried another tack.

"May I ask you a question, Doctor?"

"Certainly. What is it?"

I could tell he was already on the defensive.

"When I go to the hospital for my next checkup, do you think they'll let me have a look at my file?"

"Of course not."

"Why not? Its contents concern me intimately."

"That may be, but your file is a working file and doesn't belong to you. If you asked me to have a look at these reports"—he was holding them in his hands—"I would refuse to do so. They are mine and it's not for you to know what they contain."

"Complete trust," I said, looking at him. We both laughed.

There was nothing more I could do, and besides, what good would it do me to pry into their medical mumbo jumbo? Even if I were able to decipher it—an illegible handwriting is much practiced by doctors—my health would not be improved, and my morale might be severely strained by an incriminating word here and there.

In December, I left once again with the same cameraman to seek out my corner of Poland, this time in Perigord. Within forty-eight hours, we had experienced the gastronomic riches of the region and learned with finality that there was no hope of filming my story there with any hope of realism. The barracks we found were unusable. Even under layers of snow, if there were to be any, which was doubtful, its scattered oaks would never, no matter what the cameraman's gifts, resemble a pine forest, any more than the modest and enchanting Dordogne could stand in for the long and capricious Vistula. It became clear that we would have to find a completely different solution to our problem, or keep up the search in yet another part of France. I of course favored the latter. It's now a year later, and we're still trying to find a solution. Maybe next year. As everyone in French television knows, an author is of very questionable usefulness unless he happens to be related to the boss. An author can always wait; he's never in a hurry. If it's a matter of money, why, that's part of his profession. Besides, the libraries are full of works by famous dead authors that can be plumbed or plundered not once but many times. Live authors need only be patient; their turn will come.

A few days before Christmas, my friend came to see me to say good-bye. He had finished his treatments and had stood them well. His relief was palpable.

"The doctor says that everything's okay and he doesn't need to see me for another six months. He wrote my doctor at home to have him keep an eye on me. But it's gone!"

"Because you got it in time," I chimed in. "Now it's up to you to be sensible."

Knowing me, he could well have laughed in my face. Instead, he said with great sincerity: "Don't you worry. I don't want it to start up again."

I wasn't entirely convinced, but as he was leaving, I said: "Do me a favor, will you? Do what I've been doing these past five years. Don't hide the fact you've had cancer, that you were treated, that you're now okay. It might be of service to other people."

"You can count on me."

We slapped each other on the back like a pair of conspirators.

I love Christmas and all the memories, recent and distant, it brings back. At Christmastime, all the people I've loved and who've disappeared return to warm me with their smiles. I haven't changed; they haven't changed. They may be dead, but that doesn't mean they aren't alive somewhere else, in some other form, and no one can convince me otherwise. Then comes New Year's Eve, with mistletoe to kiss under, girls to squeeze, a birth ushered in to the din of honking horns, and "Please don't forget your postman, garbageman. . . ."

We stayed home to celebrate the last day of the unregretted old year. After a leisurely dinner, we watched to see how television would treat the event. Be merry! Have a good time! Let joy be rampant!

As the last of the twelve bells faded away, a very important person suddenly filled the screen, wished all Frenchmen a happy New Year, and as his first thought for the new year, he hoped it would bring victory over the scourge of cancer. The specificity of his hope cut through the banality usual to these occasions. And the background atmosphere of celebration gave it added impact. My wife, along with thousands of others I'm sure, was deeply moved. "He must have a big heart to think of such a thing on New Year's Eve." Then she added: "What if you wrote him? He might be able to help you."

"Perhaps."

I had solicited so many so-called generous people in my life, usually in vain, that I wasn't eager to try again. I don't mind acting humble, but being humiliated is another matter. However legitimate the cause, I don't like to look as if I were begging. "Kind sir, won't you help a poor man with cancer!" I'd rather rattle a cup in the subway. Or so I think; I haven't tried it. But a succession of dashed hopes made me need help as never before, and I had no right to pass up a chance when my wife was working her fingers to the bone so that I could go on writing. A proper middle-class family would have called me a pimp. So, for my wife's sake, I must make this effort even though it would wound my already damaged pride. Was my pride in the wrong place, perhaps?

I slept on it for a couple of nights and came to no conclusion. "What if I wrote to him?" my wife suggested one morning. I countered with the reasons, more personal than convincing, that had kept me from asking this man to order a rerun of a television program of mine that had been shown three years earlier with considerable success. To be sure, I wasn't asking him a favor. Programs made prior to mine had been rerun, some within months of their first showing.

But on second thought, my wife's solution began to make sense. It's always easier to plead someone else's cause, even when it's your husband's.

"Why not?" I said. "There's no harm in trying. But he musn't think I know anything about the letter."

So I sat down and composed the petition with just the right balance of contained emotion, dignity, and a passing allusion to the financial plight of a proud author with cancer. It struck me as perfect in every respect. My wife copied it, signed it, and dropped it in the mailbox. A month went by. With each day, our hopes dwindled. "Maybe he didn't receive it," my wife ventured, knowing perfectly well that throwing a letter in the waste basket is sound administrative procedure.

A few days later, the presentation of a literary prize to which we were invited gave her the occasion, and the luck, we thought, to meet the man she had written. With great courage, and undaunted by the people crowding around the great man, she managed to speak to him briefly. When she found me again, standing meekly near the buffet, she was radiant. I too had been surrounded and even buffeted, but not for reasons of notoriety. It was one of those rare occasions when literature feeds its practitioners, and many were taking advantage of the opportunity. Hunger in the world of letters is still endemic.

"Exactly as I thought!" she said triumphantly as we escaped the party. "He didn't get the letter and told me to write him again and put 'personal' on it."

Nothing ventured, nothing gained, so I brought forth a second and even better letter, in which "my wife" made the point that although my play had been filmed in color, it had been shown only in black and white. This time we got an answer, an unctuous, prevaricating letter with the usual regrets, written by an underling.

"I don't believe it!" my wife said. "They couldn't have read the letter. Or they didn't get the point. I'm going to write him at his home."

A third letter went out, and nothing came of that either. One disappointment is never a catastrophe when disappointments have become a habit—a habit I'm eager to break, mind you. Damocles had a sword hanging by a horsehair suspended over his head. I have a whole armory hanging over mine. From time to time, one of them drops. Horsehair isn't what it used to be. I try to soften the blow, and rush back to work, ready for the next one to fall. In this daily competition between work and the falling swords that were dropping at an accelerating rate, I had precious little time to think about my illness.

A dead hope always seems to give birth to a new one. This rule brooks few exceptions. The one born early in the year died a little before Easter. It's time was up. Three months isn't bad for a hope.

Spring was not far off, and with it came some substantial encouragement. Not the cheap encouragement of a few kind words and a handshake, but the real solid kind with which I was able to tone down some of my noisier debts, and to pay off the process server who rang my doorbell one afternoon with the insistence of a man who thought he owned the place. This is fairly rare in his difficult profession, for most of the men I have had to deal with were humane and understanding in a trade that is seldom either.

Some time ago, I was interrupted at work by the doorbell and, thinking it was someone selling soap or vacuum cleaners, I opened the door, ready to give him a piece of my mind. What was my astonishment to find three men standing outside my door! I grasped the situation in a flash. It was the process server, buttressed by a policeman and a locksmith. Never before had I faced such a deployment of forces. I must have some reputation! To be sure, I had been churlish with a process server who had interrupted a nap one day. When I learned that he only wanted to reclaim my television set for nonpayment of the tax, I was greatly relieved. To have to pay for the privilege of eating dinner to the accompaniment of a commercial boasting that it could transform my toilet into a Persian garden or keep my wife odorless for a whole day seemed to me the greatest of injustices.

For a brief moment, that is how I explained the presence of this trinity. I was soon to learn that the reinforcements were there to open my door and seize all my furniture in case I was absent. And all of it was perfectly legal. In the presence of the two walk-ons who seemed very bored with their nonspeaking roles, I exchanged a few bittersweet words with the official as he scribbled on a piece of paper and took my money. What could I do? It was three against one.

"Until next time!" I said wittily when the painful operation was over. Then, to turn my capitulation into a semblance of victory, I added: "You know, when you have cancer, you look at things with a certain detachment. . . ," which was both stupid and untrue. I'm a bad loser and anger is a poor inspiration. My exit line was a flop and, on further reflection, unworthy of me. Besides, it didn't work, for six months later, the same process server informed me he would be coming very soon if I didn't stop by his office to pay my television tax within the next three days, the tax almost doubled by the penalties already accrued for the year following the one I had already paid at such painful cost. Maybe I should have kept my mouth shut. I'm convinced that they shortened the time usually allowed. It was a mean thing to do, but understandable. With a cancerous debtor, it's best to hurry things along.

6

By the time Easter came, I barely remembered the en-
forced vacation spent in the hospital two years before. I
still went back for increasingly infrequent checkups, and
while my doctors expressed great satisfaction with my
general condition, I was not happy about the way my
face had changed shape. It seemed to flatten when I
clamped my teeth together. The corners of my mouth
dropped like a carp's, causing my chin to reach toward
my nose. So I rushed to my dentist to have him set the
matter to rights.

"Your lower jaw has retracted a bit," he said. "The
base of your prosthesis will have to be changed."

This so-called minor matter took up three whole
months and became a source of considerable contention
between my dentist and me. First it was too high, then
too low. Now we had it right. No, not quite; we'll have
to start all over again. One day I had my lower teeth, the
next day I didn't. Then, God be praised, I had them
again. This time we've really got it! No, something's
wrong. Must redo it. Now it's right. Perfect! Well, not

exactly. And we'd start all over again. This game played out with my plastic choppers required the most dogged patience. In the end, of the two players I was the more patient.

"We'll get it right in the end," I kept telling my troubled dentist when I sensed he was ready to call it quits. And in the end, we made it, thanks to his skill and my determination to give him my full support.

While this was going on, one day I'd eat my lunch, the next day I'd drink it. I scheduled my lunch engagements for the days when I had both top and bottom. Since there were occasional miscalculations, I would have to go through lunch talking with great difficulty and half a smile, the other half being at the workshop. Once again, drawing on my earlier experiences, I mumbled a brief explanation which provided me with the protection I needed.

When I had to use the telephone, I had the unarguable excuse of a poor connection, although I had no wish to falsely incriminate the telephone company. Except for this annoyance and the dullness of my diet, I had little to complain of. The frequent trips between my house and the dentist's office did wonders for my legs. The combination of frugality and exercise is a much-touted virtue. As I've said before, there is no beauty without effort.

This had been going on for two months when I happened to turn on the television set one night and caught a top ORTF figure urging all Frenchmen to leap from their chairs and run to the nearest town hall to pledge their support for the cancer division of the Institut Pasteur. The performance was a marvel of controlled persuasion, the face intent, the tie sober. Obviously, the man knew his business. "General mobilization of the nation's conscience . . . it concerns every one of us. . . ." It was a ringing appeal to our hearts and pocketbooks. Five francs a pledge. Why, it was nothing, or almost nothing, but this "almost nothing," multiplied many thousand times, could mean victory over cancer—tomorrow! During the course of the evening, the screen kept showing a rising thermometer, indicating the "magnificent" response as Frenchmen assaulted their town halls, which would remain open until midnight.

This surge was photographed in carefully selected sections of Paris. There was indeed a crowd, though smaller than the ones that hover around the pari-mutuel booths at opening times on Sundays—a question of the hour, no doubt. It had been organized like an election evening, not quite on the same scale of course. It's understandable, cancer being less important than the makeup of the Chamber of Deputies, one man's future of lesser importance than the Republic's. As the evening progressed, the gentleman on the screen began to turn the screws: "Get out of your chairs, leave your homes, your town hall isn't far, they're waiting for you, make this gesture, we beg of you. . . ."

It was a noble piece of work, but it left me cold. I instinctively distrust such well-orchestrated begging. There was one particularly false note. A young reporter, his mike in hand, was interviewing passersby to test the measure of their goodwill. Suddenly, a young woman with some kind of crippling disease seized the microphone to express, in this time of mutual aid, the anguish of people with her infirmity who could find no place in society. She was barely given time to finish her sentence. Caught by surprise, the reporter yanked the mike away from her, mumbling that she was off the subject. Her cry of despair, interrupted by this clumsy clod, left me shaken. All right, he was young and inexperienced, but still. . . . Evidently I wasn't alone, for someone came on a few moments later to apologize for the "regrettable incident." Whether she had had an accident, polio, or some birth defect was not the question; this broken woman had had the courage to go out in the dead of night to give her contribution to the fight against cancer, while I, with a pair of sturdy, well-exercised legs, sat on my ass without moving. This struggle was far more mine than hers. And if she had taken advantage of an entirely fortuitous mike thrust in her face to call attention to a disease that wasn't on the program, she was certainly within her rights. A few moments later, I was out of the house.

I walked for a while, then took an almost empty bus that left me off near the town hall. The place was all lit up as if for a celebration, although the square in front was almost deserted. A few people were sitting outside the cafés; another few coming up out of the Métro, gasping with astonishment at the blaze of light. It wasn't yet eleven o'clock; the flood of people had not materialized in my *quartier*. I walked into the town hall, alone. Alone, I left my dusty footprints on democracy's deep red carpet, and I climbed the imposing staircase, still alone. Nor was anyone following me. There wasn't a sound. It felt very strange to be alone in the midst of all this glitter. It was unreal, like a dream or a fairy tale, as if I were going to a party in my honor in a sleeping palace. What would I find at the top of the staircase? A princess?

I entered the imprssive reception room where a group of diligent citizens had sacrificed an evening to accept pledges for the eradication of cancer. Being the only client at the moment, I thought it only polite to nod and thank them with a collective smile. (There are times when I wish I were enormously rich.) Having parted with my donation, I put the pledge card in my pocket and noticed that a few latecomers were arriving. I was glad for the good people upstairs. I know how depressing it is to wait and hope when it seems unjustified.

By the end of June, I had demoted my dental problem to a matter of beneficial walks, with success a certainty. Then it came time for my quarterly visit to my hematologist. A few hours before, I picked up the X rays of my lungs I had had taken two days earlier. They didn't interest me much. As I sat having a cup of coffee in a bistro, I read the attached report of what I had taken to be a routine examination. (How easy it is to recover the expectation of good health!) As I expected, it started out well. Then things began to turn sour. "The rear mediastinum appears to have darkened, and a small adenopathy is visible on the left side." It takes talent to write that kind of rubbish. What was this blasted "mediastinum" that was getting darker, and this "adenopathy" visible on the left side? At least it was "small." And what was I doing anyway, sitting in a bistro, with my life-sized pictures spread out before me, tracking down a "mediastinum"? Being no better at deciphering X rays than tea leaves, I quickly gave up the task of interpretation.

I stuffed the pictures back in their envelope, finished my coffee, paid up, and rushed to plug up the holes in my knowledge in the book department of a large department store. I could have waited until evening; I had a sizable collection of dictionaries in my own hose. But there are thirsts for knowledge that cannot be quenched, so I ran to the nearest well. Glasses on, I started leafing through a two-volume encyclopedia: adenoid, adenoma, adenopathy. . . . Ah, "a disease of the lymphatic glands." Exactly what I expected. Two will get you three. I was ahead one. A new gland was off and running. . . .

"Can I help you, sir?"

A salesgirl was approaching me. I could have answered that I'd already helped myself once and was now looking for a second helping. But that would have been rude. She smiled; business was slow and she had plenty of time. Sorry that I was deluding her into thinking she was about to make an important sale, I took down the second volume and, turning the pages slowly like a judicious buyer, I finally arrived at "mediastinum." When I learned that it simply referred to the space between my two lungs, I closed the book and, smiling back, retreated with a lame "Thank you very much; I'll think about it," which never fooled anybody, even the most neophyte of salesgirls. I was too preoccupied to invent a more elegant leave-taking.

A gland is nothing, it's a blameless little thing. Children often have trouble with them. But they can also cause very dark thoughts in the head. Where was this one leading me? I went back over the tortuous road the other glands had led me down. The thought of doing it all over again wasn't tempting. Why did it have to find its way into my chest? Why couldn't it leave me in peace?

I wasn't very hopeful when, a little later, I handed my doctor the X rays with the accompanying note. He took the pictures but pushed the report aside.

"I don't need that. I know how to read X rays." It was a bad beginning; I was afraid I'd upset him.

"Apparently I have a small adenopathy," I ventured, boldly trying out my new vocabulary. I had a double purpose. I wanted to call his attention to it. (Look, even the greatest practitioner may be distracted at times; I was only taking a simple precaution to make sure he noticed the new trouble spot.) And, if I gave the impression that I was much better informed about my condition than in fact I was, he might take me into his confidence on a less limited basis.

"Nothing to be alarmed about," he said with a smile, and at my request, showed me where the suspect gland was on the photograph. All I could make out was a small vaguely outlined patch. Alone, I never would have had the medical insight to recognize it as a dubious gland. Besides, it had yet to prove that it was bad.

"To be on the safe side, we'll have a tomography taken," the doctor said, and started to write.

A "tomography": Now what! The treasure hunt was on again. What in God's name was a "tomography"? I already saw myself pierced through by an instrument of torture designed to analyze my adenopathy's true nature. At the risk of appearing ignorant, I asked: "What does a tomography consist of?"

I learned that it was a form of X ray that produced a series of highly selective pictures giving a precise idea of the organ's condition. I breathed easier, although a remnant of anxiety remained.

We talked a long time that day. I told him how much I loved life and how this explained my attitude to my illness. I also told him how I hoped I wouldn't be a coward when it came time to depart this life for a place which, without being a true believer, I cannot wholly dismiss. I always carry a small medallion of the Virgin my wife gave me six years ago. It helps me; in a confused way, I feel that I need its help. I'm no hero. It's difficult enough to be worthy of being called a man. As if he were echoing my thoughts, the doctor said: "It's sometimes difficult for us too. . . ."

He couldn't have given me greater proof of his esteem. I was on the verge of tears. Reformed drunk that I am, I cry easily. I smiled and discreetly placed the modest fee I owed him on his desk. No matter how many times I do it, and I should be well accustomed to it by now, I'm always acutely uncomfortable when I have to pay a doctor directly. It strikes me as incongruous and almost insulting to the doctor. Can the good someone does you be paid for in money? In the case of doctors, logically and indubitably, yes. Yet I feel ashamed when I take out a few dog-eared bills which would settle little if not accompanied by gratitude. There are debts that are unpayable. The doctor walked me to the door, and as he saw me off, he placed his hand affectionately on the back of my neck, the way you sometimes do with children, and shook my hand. He is much younger than I in years, but much wiser in the head.

I returned home reluctantly. I knew my news would worry my wife, and worry her a lot. When it's anything that concerns me, she never does things by halves. . . . Her anxiety added to mine, which of course I tried to hide, gave me a spate of days that neither work nor my trips back and forth to the dentist managed to allay. Between that first day and the day I learned the results of my tomography, I had plenty of time to wonder about my hope of not being a coward when it was time to go. Devout or not, no one is in a hurry to leave.

That word "coward" brought back the memory of my friend Laurent. We had known each other in prison camp—we were there for "attempted escape"—and had stayed together until we parted in the middle of a potato field in the Ukraine, momentarily Germanified. Then our itineraries diverged. Very tall, solidly built, an easy talker with a biting but never cruel wit, he had the style and brio of a Gascon and needed lessons in courage from nobody. About a year after the end of the war, we met again in Paris, and the first thing he told me was: "You should be dead by now, you know. The condition you were in when I left you, you didn't have a chance in a million of coming out of it alive."

When I was having my first operation, I got in touch with Laurent, and he came to see me as soon as my nose was unplugged. "You know," he said, "if I ever have cancer, I'll meet it squarely, the way you're doing."

At the beginning of December, he called me to tell me he was having chest X rays taken. A few days before Christmas, he called me again.

"I've got cancer, but mine is a bigger bitch than yours."

His "little thing" had been an excruciating pain in the shoulder which hit him as he was lifting a barbell in a gym where he went to keep in shape. He thought it was just a strained muscle. It wasn't. "I'm going to have my operation after the holidays," he said. "It's wiser. I know doctors. . . ." He loved to crack jokes, but I knew he could be trusted. He had confidence in his doctors. But he didn't have my luck.

"Now you," he told me affably just before his operation, "you could go under the knife two or even three times. It wouldn't bother you. Your temperament can take it. Not me: once is it."

His personal forecast was severe but carefully calculated. He would never die a loser. And with my affection for him and everything that bound us together, I knew he'd come through. He was made for victory.

Well, the cards weren't stacked that way. Things went from bad to worse. The hospital where he was having the operation turned out not to have the necessary equipment, and they had to rush him to another hospital in the middle of the night. His life hung in the balance for several weeks, his big body artificially kept alive while his soul wandered off, God knows where. When he finally and miraculously came out of his long and heartrending coma, I was allowed to visit him. He greeted me with a big smile. "You see, I've come back from the banks of the Styx. The terrible boatman wanted no part of me."

His "trip" hadn't changed him, and I believed with all my soul that, in spite of the prognosis that gave him only a few months' remission, he would give his doctors the lie. At the start of his convalescence, which he spent in a very comfortable retreat outside Paris, he seemed to my joy to be giving as good as he got. His splendid appetite, long the subject of admiration and astonishment, was back. "You wouldn't find a place like this for twenty thousand old francs," he said with amazement. "And when you think that it doesn't cost me a sou! . . ." And he sang the praises of our Social Security which ill-informed people so love to criticize. When his stay at the home was over, he returned to Paris. Despite all the care and affection lavished on him, he quickly went downhill. One day, when I went to visit him, I greeted him with a jaunty "So, Laurent, how are things today?"

He stopped me dead in my tracks. "No! Not from you!" Looking me straight in the eye, he added: "Also, will you please tell your boys to stop asking how I am each time they telephone."

He knew better than I did that he was going to die, and he was making it very clear that he wanted me to cut the crap. Since there was nothing more to say on that subject, we talked of other things. That was five years ago.

I thought about him as I lay stretched out under the X-ray machine.

"Hold your breath. Now let it out. Wait. Don't move."

I felt as if my fate were attached to that prying eye, jerking and throbbing as it explored my mediastinum. Between the endless pictures, I contemplated the tiled ceiling. I felt like a turtle on its back but without the freedom to wiggle my legs. Had I tried, it would have been considered conduct unbecoming. It's been a long time since I had the clumsy grace of an infant, and it wouldn't do to be caught playing with my toes.

The next day, I learned that everything was entirely normal and that I could dismiss my gland from my thoughts.

With that worry behind me, I once again concentrated on my work and the continuing fittings at my dentist's. By the end of July, we had it licked so far as chewing was concerned. As for my speech, that had to be watched like a hawk. If I spoke a little too fast, even I wasn't sure what I was saying. For my friends, it was a problem both of translation and of protection from my joyful spluttering. A new prosthesis produces a great deal of saliva, and it behooves the wearer to control his verbal delivery. Why did God make me such a talker!

I paid my dentist, forgot everybody else, and we left for the seashore. Summer arrived with us, one of the most beautiful within memory. I rediscovered, as always with the same delight, our old house behind its iron fence which every year became more dilapidated, and where, more than anyplace else, I felt at home. Even the winter burglars who had worked our house couldn't dampen my joy. Three clocks, a sword, and a few nick-nacks—so what? We reported it at the police station, and it was filed away with hundreds like it. Winters are long in summer resorts. I tried to comfort my wife for the losses: "Just wait until we're rich!" We put things back in order and concentrated on being happy.

One of my first visits was to my friend at the bistro. I knew he was well, but I wanted to see for myself.

"You need some color on your face," he said as we drank our traditional glass to friendship, his water, mine a well-diluted mildly alcoholic apéritif.

"Here's to you!" he said, clicking his glass against mine. Then he added in a voice loud enough for all to hear: "Yes, sir, we're buddies more than ever now, aren't we! We've both had cancer, and we both had the same doctor."

It was very gratifying to see that he was doing what I'd asked him to. And it wasn't easy when you ran a café where old retired people came to linger over their drinks or play cards in a corner. These good souls don't like having their prejudices tampered with, and they don't like people talking lightly about death. And cancer is death. Try to tell them otherwise and they'll give you a dirty look. Not all of them, of course, but many, and some of them quite young. Stubbornness is not confined to the old, any more than a youthful heart is the exclusive attribute of twenty-year-olds.

As I write these elementary truths, my mind goes back to a story that an old friend and unrepentant bohemian told me about an experience he'd been through. He'd been sitting quietly having a drink on a bistro terrace when a group of teenagers on noisy motorbikes staged a rodeo right in front of him. Furious at the racket, he got up to give them a piece of his mind. "If you don't stop this immediately, I'll knock your heads together!"

One of the boys stopped, looked at him with more pity than anger, and said: "You poor old bastard!"

My friend observed to me: "The kid was right."

Coming from a man near eighty, I found this charming. He was always happiest with younger people anyway. It was too bad that the Lord had to claim him last year. We miss his youth. When we talk about him, which is often, it's always with a smile. He loved life too much to let himself become old. It was a blow not to find him in the places where we used to meet, but I certainly wasn't going to look him up in his grave. A cemetery is no place to find your friends. When I wander among the tombstones, as I sometimes do, it's in order to imagine the kinds of lives these unknown people lived, especially when a new name has been added to a family grave, opening up possibilities of reunions and loves resumed. Bones leave me cold. It's in my heart that my friends are buried.

The only cloud in the otherwise glorious summer weather was the implacable problem of my denture. A local lady dentist took over from her Paris colleague. In two sessions, with a few well aimed applications of her grinding wheel, she managed to get rid of the last few painful rough edges. It is said that the famous orator Demosthenes filled his mouth with pebbles to improve his sloppy diction. I had enough impediments in mine without having to add pebbles. I resorted to the much easier method of starting with the simplest words and moving on to the more difficult, always articulating with the greatest care. "I am speaking better, I am speaking better, I am speaking better. . . ." I don't know how many times I repeated this lie before it began to approximate the pale shadow of truth. I still have a long way to go, but I'm not worried. I'm in no hurry. It will come. And if it never comes back completely, that won't bother me either.

I know of few joys greater than waking up and watching the birth of a new day in my garden. I usually get up before the rest of the family, and I savor a pleasure that wouldn't be the same if I weren't alone. Standing barefoot on the cool earth, alone in the first rays of the sun, admiring my rampageous fig tree that I prune unskillfully every year, I take a deep breath and look around me with the fleeting certainty that everything is well with me, my life, and my destiny, and that I am at the center of a universe that belongs entirely to me. Then, because I am not a hopeless egotist, I open the gate of my kingdom, take a few steps down the street as it slowly comes back to life, and stop at the intersection. From there I can see the signal station, a source of local pride on a par with our *chaudrée*, our native fish soup, and observe the direction of the wind and hence what weather to expect. Sometimes I watch the wanderings of an inquisitive dog who has slipped his leash, wave at the baker's wife hawking her hot bread, or greet a neighbor as she opens her window, and return home bringing with me our battered garbage pail. On the morning we left, the garbage truck took the poor old recycled laundry tub off along with its contents. It must have met its end in the truck's grinding jaws. Walking on the wet sand, the tiny waves breaking over my feet like timid caresses, I feel the same sensation of purity and youth I experience in my tiny garden.

Toward the end of August, after the inevitable trip to Paris for the monthly perfusion, a camera-toting friend caught me for posterity standing on the beach, surrounded by colorful beach umbrellas and young things broiling their bodies in the sun. With one arm raised to the skies, I look like a prophet. I adore that photograph and show it at the slightest opportunity. I look exceptionally good half-naked.

And by September, I was making real progress with my elocution. I could exchange a few words in the street without emitting gibberish, but I still showered the countryside with the precision of an old watering can. People on either side of me are as vulnerable as those in front. My tongue is adapting itself, but it still plays tricks on me.

Toward the end of the month, the weather was so fine that I decided to put off my next perfusion in Paris for a week. Each year I find it harder to leave behind my summer ways and my affection for the country I can claim as my own only during the summer months. The people are no better or worse than anywhere else, but I love them with all their faults because we belong to the same race. We are always more indulgent toward those who resemble us. My neighbors think they know everything. Their critical functions are highly developed, their talk is loud and glib, they love to invent caustic names for the various characters around town. I'm sure that by now they've christened me "Chicken Neck," which I'm fully prepared to take in stride. My photograph happens to be taken full face, and my neck is barely noticeable. Of course, it's not in perfect focus, but still. . . .

So we returned to Paris at the last moment possible. Everybody at the hospital remarked on how well I looked. The nose and throat doctor, the X-ray technician, the nurses all seemed glad to see me in such good health. At home, things were less rosy. I kept repeating "They're not going to get me," but "they" took in a larger and larger segment of my life. Creditors, leaking plumbing, dunning letters, the noise of the floor waxer upstairs, the cloying phone calls ("Listen pal, do you think you could possibly . . ."), the dog downstairs bewailing its solitude. For all my clever calculations, as I plug one hole, I make another. But I wasn't going to let them spoil my life. Up to now, they had tried to, but they had failed.

The only thing "they" succeeded in doing was to raise my blood pressure. By the end of the month, it was wavering between 220 and 230, which is really too high. When my hematologist was informed of this inflation—in tune with the times—he summoned me posthaste.

He received me warmly as always, and leafed through the reports of the blood tests made before each perfusion.

"What about the October perfusion?" he asked with some asperity. That made me angry. After all, I am a very conscientious patient.

"I had the perfusion, only I won't be getting the report until next time." And I added, as I was putting my pants back on, "Don't worry. I'm not keeping anything from you."

My doctor laughed. Seeing that he was back in good humor, I decided to seize the opportunity to ask a few questions about my future:

"About these perfusions, Doctor. Could you tell me what stage I'm at in my treatments?"

"Why, certainly."

"Will you be completely honest?"

"Of course." (What a liar!)

He glanced through my files for a moment and announced flatly:

"You're around fifty percent done."

In other words, I was halfway through, which therefore meant another two and a half years. Christ! And I thought I was almost through! I also had the vivid memory of a stormy session in his office a year and a half before when he said, "Why are you stopping treatments when you're eighty percent through?"

Clearly, we had different views about time. His was naturally much less rigid than that of his patients, who, come what may, had to go through hell every twenty-eight days. I would have bet my last sou that he had no recollection of those earlier percentages, which I'm sure he arrived at only to calm my apprehensions. He knew me better now. And I knew him better too. I saw no point in getting involved in useless arguments about numbers. His version would always take precedence.

"Lie down, please."

He took my blood pressure: 190 on one arm, 150 on the other. That was something new. I didn't know that I was asymmetrical in this area too. After a thorough going-over with his stethoscope, I got dressed. When I returned, he had worked out a program of blood tests to challenge the most dedicated lab assistant, a request for X rays of my kidneys, and a cystography, a new word in my lexicon.

"I'm writing to a cardiologist-friend of mine. He'll have you come to his hospital when he has the results of these tests."

Then he proceeded to dictate a letter to his friend, including several details about the interesting specimen he was sending his way.

". . . he was at one time given to a certain. . . ."

"Intemperance," I said with a smile, having correctly guessed that this was the term he was looking for to inform his colleague of my old vice. (It is wise to cooperate with your doctor if you want the best care.)

"Intemperance," he repeated, thanking me out of the corner of his eye, and ended the letter with a couple of flattering remarks before professing his undying friendship, etc.

The tests brought forth nothing unusual, nor did the X rays, but there was a small something that the cardiologist picked up later.

So, early one morning, I presented myself at yet another hospital. By now well practiced in the ways of hospital waiting rooms, I had come with enough reading matter for a long morning, with a crossword puzzle held in reserve. The usual preliminary steps: pleasant reception, smiles all around, pay at the cashier's window, make out the form, thanks back and forth, a nod at those already waiting, and I sat down to my reading. Like a waltz, the consultation involved three steps.

First step, one hour of reading, followed by the electrocardiogram. My name was called out; "Good morning, strip to the waist, please"; "Lie down, please"; wires connected me to a machine. Light humming noise. The machine traced a pattern on a ribbon of paper, then spewed out the revealing rhythm of one instant of my life. How was it? Good or bad? I'd love to know what my heart told him. Now it was over and I was unplugged. Clothes back on, thank you and good-bye, and my return to the community of anxious faces. Cardiac patients usually have anxious faces. Not me. In spite of my blood pressure and the sound of my heart beating like an old pump, I thought it unlikely that my heart would join my other problems.

Second step: another hour of reading, and my name was called out again. I found myself in the hands of two students. They couldn't have been much older than my sons, and it pleased me to facilitate their task. I told them what I'd had, what treatments. One of them took it all down, then we moved to the matter at hand. "Strip to the waist, please, and take off your shoes." They weighed me. Okay there. Then they measured me. Not so good. I had lost almost half an inch since military service. What had happened to that half-inch? I couldn't believe that a man wore down at the feet. I asked the young man to measure me again. Same result. I had to accept the cruel evidence that the years were taking their toll. To a man who is no giant, the loss of a half-inch can be disturbing, but there are new and modish ways to make up the loss. The current style among the young, and others too, sadly, is to wear platform soles. If the girls are going to totter on stilts, then their males, in order not to be dominated, have to do likewise. Now, I happen to be of medium size, and I look at life from a height that suits me very well. "Lie down, please. . . ." They took my blood pressure and looked perplexed. And a thorough going-over with a stethoscope failed to reveal the mystery of my "dissymmetry." We laughed, and I put my clothes back on.

I was on the crossword puzzle when my name rang out again. Third step. An affable and courteous cardiologist gave me a detailed examination, for the benefit as well of a group of attentive students. Among his conclusions, dictated on the spot to my hematologist, I remember only that I had a sound heart—which I had never doubted but it was nice to hear all the same—and a "stenosis of the left subclavian vein." I learned later that this meant a narrowing of an artery, nothing serious. A simple treatment would normalize my blood pressure. He ended his letter to my doctor with gracious thanks for entrusting his patient to him, etc.

7

It's now seven years since my "little thing" started off on its adventure. As I said at the beginning, this story is my story. And I repeat, I have not set myself up as an example because not everybody has had my luck, and no two cases are ever exactly alike.

I had several reasons for writing my story. Not the least of them was a chance encounter with a young friend who also practices the perilous profession of writing. When I described to him what I had in mind, he said, "How lucky you are to have such a subject!"

I may be wrong, but I thought I detected a hint of envy in his remark. I liked the idea that I was the object of professional jealousy. I admit that I'm shameless. I pick up anything and everything I think might be useful to my morale. It's a form of personal paramedical treatment, and the doctors who took care of me and still do, happily with more sophisticated therapies, are well aware of its important and probably irreplaceable value. So, in all honesty, I cannot take full credit for my fight against the terror of cancer that all levels of society cultivate with such morbid delight. It's as if people actually enjoyed frightening themselves.

Whenever a journalist or writer wants to pull out all the stops to describe some ghastly catastrophe, fatal suffering, or indescribable horror, the first word he hits on is "cancer." It's the shock word par excellence to galvanize his readers. "The poverty in our ghettos is spreading like cancer"; or "The automobile is fast becoming a cancer." The writers in these two cases used the word because they felt it described the alarming proportions of the problem so aptly, never giving a thought to the disease itself or the diabolical effect of the word on many of their readers. Without meaning to, they were making cancer even more frightening. Why this need to identify everything evil in modern life as a cancer? In the scale of human fears, it has taken the place of the plague, cholera, and smallpox. Compared with cancer, syphilis is a disease for choirboys.

Therein may lie our hope. Perhaps in the not too distant future, our descendants will use the word "cancer" as casually as we now use "pest." Today we say to a small child, "Scram, you little pest!" In the future, we'll say: "You're going to get it, you little cancer!" It's the fate of scourges to end up as merely derisory. This is how man gets his revenge against the things he dreads most. The other night in the metro, I was watching a group of teenagers kidding around and cuffing each other, when one of them suddenly clutched his side and cried out in mock pain: "Ouch! You rat, you hit my cancer!" Everybody laughed, including me.

But this is a rare occurrence. Little by little, in a thousand different ways, cancer has become a traumatizing word to the point where, in spite of daily scientific progress, the word is taboo. Few doctors, nurses, technicians, or therapists will use the word in front of a patient even when his cancer is one of those known to be curable. They are encouraged in their silence by the patient's relatives: "Above all, Doctor, don't let him know he has it. He couldn't bear it!" It's well intentioned, to be sure, but it also indicates a low opinion of the person involved. Why assume that he is incapable of facing the truth? Surrounding him with a web of lies makes him fearful and a coward. Unless he is a complete fool, he'll have his own suspicions about the "benign tumor," the recurring polyp, the abnormal growth. And most patients know enough about the various forms of cancer treatment to guess why they are following this one or that. So he has two choices: either he will play the ostrich and refuse to face facts, or he will leap to the conclusion that "if they haven't told me anything, it's because I'm a goner." From then on, each second of his life is the countdown before his lift-off to eternity.

The inevitable question, so often argued, for which there is no satisfactory answer, is, "When cancer is diagnosed, should the patient be told?" In Italy, apparently, the patient is told nothing. In France, the family is told. In the United States, the patient has a right to the complete truth. No one of these three solutions is ideal. There are more than a hundred forms of cancer, some curable, some less so, and others which aren't now but may be so tomorrow. And the question solicits as many answers as there are patients.

So I think it's high time people stopped using cancer as a scare word, the fatal disease before which the whole world trembles. And its verbal derivatives: "You musn't eat this, it's carcinogenic"; "Don't breathe that, it's carcinogenic"; "Don't use . . ." From one so-called carcinogenic product to the next, you soon get to the point where you deprive yourself of everything that makes life livable, a life already imperiled by all those marvelous electronic brains with their notorious human insensibility.

Mind you, I'm not against progress. I am only disturbed by what is often perpetrated in its name. A few weeks ago, I went to the process server, whom I've already mentioned, to pay my television tax. I wanted to spare him yet another burdensome trip. As I left his office in a somewhat unsavory part of town (not his fault, I'm sure), I turned down a busy street that led toward a boulevard to catch a bus to my next appointment. As I was walking, I glanced down the narrow picturesque side streets condemned to disappear in the name of renovation. I'm not much given to nostalgia, and I'm ready to admit that crumbling, unsanitary buildings should come down. But when I see what is put up in their place, I become concerned. Concrete monsters without souls, built for maximum profit and rentability, places where it will become increasingly difficult to know, understand, and love one another. Developers are not much given to sentiment. My thoughts were interrupted by the realization that although the bulldozers had already eaten up several houses and were on their way to a new feast, the prostitutes had not disappeared. In fact, there were lots of them. Given the time of day, they must be servicing the early lunch crowd.

Seeing them there, I suddenly decided to put into execution an idea I'd been harboring for a long time. Girding up my courage, I said: "The next one is it." It takes guts to accost a prostitute at high noon in full view of the midday crowd. I hadn't gone ten feet when I noticed a superb amazon, outrageously made up, and exposing

with arrogance the billowing charms of her powerful fe-
maleness. A sidewalk monument! It was too much. I
wasn't man enough. If she happened to take offense at
what I had in mind, she could reduce me to putty. So I
prudently continued on my way as if I hadn't seen her,
which, even for the shortsighted mole I am, was virtually
impossible. Once out of danger, I flailed myself for my
cowardice and, determined not to give in for "moral"
reasons, turned down a narrow little-traveled street.

Luck smiled on me. Sheltered under the overhang of
an old porch, a young thing was cowering like a small
cornered animal. When she saw me looking her over, she
gave me a timid smile and, without saying a word,
opened her coat to reveal two small, white, well-rounded
breasts. She must have been new at the trade. I walked up
to her.

"May I ask you a question?"

She stopped smiling, and her expression changed to
distrust. "What is it?"

"Would you go upstairs with a client who had cancer?"

"Sure, why not?"

It was as simple as that. I had the proof I wanted: it
wasn't contagious, it didn't harm anyone else. (Professional conscience is the artisan's pride.) I thanked the girl
and left, wishing her the best of luck.

A little later, I asked the same question of a gorgeous
specimen in one of the better sections of town. She was
standing next to a car, jiggling her car keys. Her answer
was identical. I even had some trouble making a polite
getaway, for the lady was very desirable and seemed
eager to drive me off toward heaven knows what sexual
delights. With the price of gas being what it is, I was
afraid it might be beyond my slender means. But I had
what I wanted, and from the lips of women who were

prepared to put it to the test virtually on the spot. I've always had great respect for public girls, more than for most public men.

I would also like to say a few things about doctors in general. I myself have had only the best of doctors, to whom I'm forever grateful. But from what I hear, I've been very lucky. For me, there is no such thing as a bad doctor; a bad doctor is not a doctor at all. As in no other profession, the man who has chosen to heal his fellow-man is under the obligation to resist weakness in all its forms. But we pay a price for maintaining their superiority, and for preserving the distances between them and those of us on "the other side." The profession's moral obligations, medical deontology, have evolved through long experience and a vast accretion of knowledge. But I who belong to "the other side" would like to sound a small warning: we patients are perhaps not as stupid as we once were. It's not our fault; progress has done it to us.

While doctors try to resist the desires common to all men, they are subjected to the constant additional temptation of believing they are what their patients would have them be. Not God, to be sure—that place is already taken. But something like him. Unfortunately, that is not possible. To have the knowledge to cure is one thing; to exercise power is something else again. The nearest thing a doctor has to divinity, if it exists at all, is the love of humanity that determined his choice of career in the first place, his conscience which is constantly assailed by the crushing responsibilities he must bear, and his humility in the face of the unknown. That is a lot. The same goes for the nurses, therapists, technicians, orderlies. All these people often do thankless tasks under impossible conditions, yet never become robots and are always ready with a smile, a gesture, or a single word that may do more good than all the treatments in the medical arsenal. Other patients may not have experienced this, but perhaps they weren't seeking it, or didn't deserve it.

Having promised myself that I would be honest from beginning to end, I now feel obliged to explain the least attractive motive for writing this book. I could be a hypocrite and pretend that I did it to render a service to humanity, and some would probably believe me. The idea that this long journey through my recent past might be of some help to someone else was not totally absent from my mind. But there are also personal reasons already hinted at many times.

Writing is my trade. And, as I've made no pains to hide, I have financial worries to spare. I am very anxious to be rid of my debts. About five years ago, I was "invited" to appear before the Magistrate's Court in my *arrondissement* concerning a matter of an unpaid bill for my son's boarding school in the country. To explain my prolonged default, I mentioned my straitened circumstances and the mitigating fact that I had written my creditor several times to tell him that I had not forgotten my debt and that I would pay him fully and with interest as soon as I could.

"You see, sir," I said as I concluded, "I mean well."

From the heights of his throne, the judge let go with a blow that would have felled a much more hardened criminal than I.

"Sir," he said sternly, "a man who owes money never means well."

Christ! In that case, I had seldom meant well during my long life. If his pronouncement were true, I would have to revise my whole conception of life and friendship. Was he right? Had the value I placed on money been inadequate? I understood that the reason I had lost my richer friends was because I owed them money. Luckily, I'd been able to keep the less rich. They continued to remain my friends and, from the time of my first operation, expressed their generosity with both their hearts and their pocketbooks. They had confidence in me, and now it's time I proved that their confidence wasn't misplaced.

Some will accuse me of trying to make money out of cancer. Well, I'm not the first. Besides, my cancer belongs to me, and I have every right to sell it if I like. I'm not selling anybody else's. Nowadays, when people are making money out of anything and everything, why can't I try to make money out of what is mine? Obviously, a publisher would prefer that I'd escaped from prison, was an archbishop's son, the owner of a bordello, a transvestite, or maybe an assassin. My "adventure" would then have the gamy smell that makes best-sellers. Too bad; that is not where my luck lay.

In the end, it was for my own sake that I communed with myself at such length. In telling my story, I hoped to come to grips with my fear. When the moment came, I hoped to have the courage that, had I been a believer, faith would have given me. I've tried to find this faith, I'm not ashamed to admit it. I suspect it's somewhere, but it escapes me. So I've had to invent my own God; the God of my childhood had been spoiled for me by the shameless demagoguery of those who represent his church. The man who was nailed to the cross gave a new meaning to men's hopes when he said: "The Kingdom of God is within you." I know even less about theology than medicine, which is why I am able to believe that by constantly demanding more of myself, as Christ did, I may someday find God. In the meantime, while awaiting the blessed encounter, I have devised a number of formulas to keep me going. "Love life and don't fear death." "Should I die tomorrow, even if God has not given me faith, he will surely hold out his hand."

And I've had the ultimate justification for my confidence in the future. I was born on Friday the thirteenth, under the sign of the Virgin. Using my birth date, I once bet a big triple on the horses. I won. My neighbors have never forgotten it. We were rich for a whole month!